50 Barbara O'Neill Inspired Herbal
Home Remedies & Natural Medicine.

Volume 1

www.abetteryoueveryday.com

Over 350 Barbara O'Neill Inspired Herbal Healing Home Remedies & Natural Medicine

Holistic Approach to Organic Health, Natural Cures and Nutrition for Sustaining Body and Mind Healing

Volume 1

By Margaret Willowbrook

USA

2024

TABLE OF CONTENTS

GLIMPSE INTO THE CHAPTERS AHEAD

In the serene embrace of nature, Margaret Willowbrook found her calling. Inspired by the teachings of Barbara O'Neill, a renowned figure in herbal healing, Margaret embarks on a journey to share this wisdom. An anecdote of transformation, where a simple herb alleviated a chronic ailment, sets the stage. This book is not just about plants and remedies; it's about reconnecting with the healing powers of nature, a principle deeply rooted in O'Neill's teachings.

Chapter 1: Foundations of Herbal Medicine.

Dive into the world of herbal medicine as taught by Barbara O'Neill. Margaret begins with a captivating real-life example showcasing the efficacy of herbal understanding. Delve into the properties of various herbs, learning about their healing benefits and how to safely gather and prepare them. This chapter isn't just informative; it's a doorway to the ancient wisdom of natural healing.

Chapter 2: Herbal Safety and Contraindications.

Safety is paramount in herbal medicine. This chapter discusses the protocols emphasized by O'Neill, integrating a reflective segment on understanding herbal safety. Margaret goes into potential side effects and interactions of herbs. Special precautions for specific conditions and medications are also outlined, ensuring a comprehensive understanding of herbal safety.

Chapter 3: Herbal Remedies for Common Ailments.

Enter the heart of herbal healing with detailed recipes for treating common ailments. Each is introduced with a story or case study, illustrating the real-life impact of O'Neill's remedies. Learn about preparation techniques, dosages, and frequencies. This chapter is a practical guide, rich in anecdotes and wisdom, bringing the power of herbs to your fingertips.

Chapter 4: Specialized Herbal Treatments.

Focusing on specific conditions, this chapter offers herbal recipes based on O'Neill's extensive knowledge. Learn how to combine herbs for enhanced effects and tailor treatments to individual needs. Interactive elements invite readers to consider how these treatments can be personalized, making the chapter a participatory experience.

Chapter 5: Holistic Herbal Regimens.

Explore the creation of holistic treatment plans. Understand how different remedies work in synergy, a concept central to O'Neill's teachings. This chapter emphasizes the balance of herbal treatments with lifestyle changes, advocating for a comprehensive approach to health and well-being.

Chapter 6: Herbal Detoxification and Cleansing.

Margaret guides you through the methods of herbal detox and cleansing as practiced by O'Neill. Learn about the role of detoxification in holistic healing and safe practices for conducting herbal detoxification. Actionable steps at the end of the chapter provide a practical guide for starting your detox journey.

Chapter 7: Long-term Management of Chronic Conditions.

This chapter addresses managing chronic diseases with herbal remedies. Incorporate lifestyle and dietary considerations into your regimen. Inspirational success stories demonstrate the real-world application of these methods, providing hope and practical advice for those dealing with long-term health conditions.

Chapter 8: Women's and Men's Health.

Address gender-specific health issues through herbal remedies. Discover herbal solutions for hormonal balance and reproductive health, supported by real-life examples. This chapter not only informs but also empowers, providing targeted solutions for both women and men.

Chapter 9: Children's Herbal Remedies.

Margaret introduces safe and effective herbal treatments for children. Learn how to adjust dosages and formats for pediatric use and navigate common misconceptions about children's herbal care. This chapter is a valuable resource for parents seeking natural health solutions for their little ones.

Chapter 10: Mental and Emotional Well-being.

Focusing on mental health, this chapter explores herbs for stress relief and overall mental well-being. It offers methods for improving mental and emotional wellness. Reflective questions and exercises help apply these teachings to personal mental health scenarios, making this chapter a journey of self-discovery.

Chapter 11: Seasonal Herbal Remedies.

Adapt your herbal treatments with the changing seasons. Learn season-specific wellness tips, reflecting O'Neill's understanding of nature's rhythms. A seasonal anecdote or story aligns with O'Neill's teachings, bringing a personal touch to this chapter.

Chapter 12: Incorporating Herbs into Daily Life.

Learn to integrate herbs into your daily routine. This chapter offers a clear plan for readers to start incorporating herbs into their daily life. It's not just about healing; it's about enhancing daily wellness through nature.

Chapter 13: Sustainable and Ethical Sourcing of Herbs.

Margaret emphasizes sourcing herbs sustainably and ethically, respecting nature. This chapter includes a discussion on the importance of sustainability in herbal practice, urging readers to consider the impact of their choices on the environment and local communities.

Chapter 14: Herbal Preservation and Storage.

Discover techniques for preserving and storing herbs, ensuring their potency and effectiveness. This chapter provides practical tips and homework for implementing these techniques, turning theory into practice.

Chapter 15: Herbal First Aid Kit.

Build a basic kit of herbal remedies for immediate needs. This chapter offers a quick reference guide for emergency treatments and a compelling story about the importance of a herbal first aid kit.

Chapter 16: Empowering Yourself through Herbal Knowledge.

Finally, equip yourself with tools and resources for continuing education in herbal medicine. Reflecting O'Neill's commitment to lifelong learning, this chapter encourages experimentation with herbal recipes and provides a call to action for further study and application.

Conclusion.

Margaret Willowbrook concludes with a summary of O'Neill's teachings, encouraging readers to embrace the power of nature. The final reflections draw on O'Neill's wisdom, leaving readers inspired and empowered on their journey to natural health.

Last Chapter: Detailed recipes for treating common conditions inspired by O'Neill's remedies.

The book concludes with a comprehensive last chapter with over 300 detailed Recipes for Treating Common Conditions, making it an invaluable resource for anyone who did get this book.

References.

Attention!

Before you dive into this captivating book, we have an exclusive offer just for you! A fantastic FREE Bonus:

Get Your Ready-to-Print Herbal Reference Guide Bonuses!

Remedy Recipes (6 pages)   **Herbal First Aid** (4 pages)   **Herb Directory** (6 pages)

EXPLORE A VARIETY OF NATURAL, EASY-TO-PREPARE REMEDY RECIPES FOR DAILY HEALTH NEEDS, SPANNING STRESS RELIEF TO IMMUNE SUPPORT.   ACCESS DETAILED HERBAL SOLUTIONS FOR COMMON HEALTH ISSUES, PROVIDING NATURAL EMERGENCY CARE ALTERNATIVES.   DELVE INTO AN EXTENSIVE DIRECTORY OF MEDICINAL HERBS, COMPLETE WITH USES, BENEFITS, AND PREPARATION TIPS.

These printable guides, crafted after extensive research and dedication, offer quick, easy access to a wealth of herbal remedies, recipes, and first aid information. Designed for fast reference, they cover everything from specific herbs in our 'Herb Directory', to swift recipes in 'Remedy Recipes', and practical emergency care in 'Herbal First Aid'. Though we plan to sell them separately in the future, we're currently offering these guides for free as our appreciation for your book purchase, as a way of saying thank you and adding extra value to your reading experience.

For instant delivery, simply chat with our Facebook bot via the link below or scan the accompanying QR code.

http://tinyurl.com/Herbalbonuses

Alternatively, you can request the guides by emailing us at: info@abetteryoueveryday.com.
Enjoy your reading and these additional resources!

FOREWORD

My dear readers,

As you gently open the pages of " Over 350 Barbara O'Neill Inspired Herbal Healing Home Remedies & Natural Medicine," please know that you are not just launching into a book, but embarking on a journey very dear to my heart. This book, lovingly assembled, is not merely a compendium of herbal remedies; it is a vessel carrying the profound essence of nature's healing wisdom, a wisdom that has graced my life and which I now share with you.

Brought to light by the teachings of the remarkable Barbara O'Neill, a guiding light in natural health, this book is my humble offering to you. I do not proclaim myself a specialist; rather, I see myself as a fellow traveler on the path to understanding the bounty of nature. It is my deepest hope that the wisdom shared here, a blend of Barbara's teachings and my own learning, will guide and comfort you as it has me.

As we journey together through these pages, I invite you to join me with an open heart and mind. Embrace the possibilities nature unfolds, and let each piece of advice be a step towards better health and a deeper harmony with the world around us.

I must ask for your kindness and understanding as you read. This book, a labor of love, is my first attempt to collate the wealth of knowledge I've encountered. If you find any errors or have suggestions, I warmly welcome your feedback. Your insights will be invaluable in making this a living, evolving guide.

With all my warmth and kindness,

Margaret Willowbrook

Author Introduction

Welcome, dear readers, to " Over 350 Barbara O'Neill Inspired Herbal Healing Home Remedies & Natural Medicine." As you embark on this journey through the pages of this book, I extend my hand to you, not as an expert or a guru, but as a fellow traveler who has walked the path of discovery and awe in the realm of natural healing. This book is a heartfelt endeavor to bring together the teachings of Barbara O'Neill, a beacon of wisdom in herbal healing, and my own experiences and insights gathered along the way.

The Genesis of a Healing Journey

My journey into the world of natural remedies began many years ago, under the quiet, watchful eyes of the towering trees and whispering herbs in my garden. Like many of you, I was once reliant on the quick fixes and promises of modern medicine, seeking relief but finding only temporary solace. It was in nature's embrace that I found true healing, not just for the body, but for the soul as well.

Barbara O'Neill's teachings were a revelation to me. Her approach to health and wellness, deeply rooted in the natural world, resonated with my own beliefs and experiences. She taught not just about herbs and their uses, but about a way of life; a life where one is in sync with the rhythms of nature, respectful of the body's innate wisdom, and mindful of the holistic nature of wellbeing. This book is my humble attempt to bring her teachings to a wider audience, woven together with my personal narrative and understanding.

A Living Conversation

This book is more than just a static collection of knowledge. It's a living conversation between you, me, and the natural world. As you read, I invite you to interact with the content, to reflect on your own experiences, and to apply the insights in a way that resonates with your personal journey.

I must also ask for your understanding and patience. As much as I have strived to ensure accuracy and comprehensiveness, there may be imperfections and areas for growth. I welcome your feedback and insights, as they are invaluable in making this a living, evolving guide.

Embracing Nature's Wisdom

As we conclude this introduction, I want to thank you for choosing to embark on this journey with me. My hope is that "Over 350 Barbara O'Neill Inspired Herbal Healing Home Remedies & Natural Medicine." becomes more than just a book on your shelf; that it becomes a companion on your path to wellness, a source of comfort, and a testament to the incredible healing power of nature.

So, dear readers, let us begin this journey together. Let us learn, heal, and grow in the gentle embrace of nature's wisdom.

With all my love and best wishes,

Margaret Willowbrook

Introduction of the Book

Welcome to a journey of rediscovery and healing, a journey that bridges the wisdom of the past with the needs of the present. This journey is not just about herbs and their properties; it's about embracing a holistic way of life, deeply rooted in the rhythms of nature. "Over 350 Barbara O'Neill Inspired Herbal Healing Home Remedies & Natural Medicine." is a heartfelt invitation to explore the world of natural healing, guided by the teachings of Barbara O'Neill and my personal experiences with herbal medicine.

In writing this book, I have sought to create a space where wisdom, tradition, and modern understanding coalesce. It is a space where the teachings of Barbara O'Neill, a luminary in natural health, illuminate the path toward holistic wellbeing. This journey is as much about understanding the herbs themselves as it is about embracing a lifestyle that aligns with the natural world.

The Inspiration Behind the Journey

At the heart of this book is a profound respect and admiration for Barbara O'Neill. Her approach to natural health, characterized by a deep understanding of the body's natural rhythms and an unwavering faith in the healing power of nature, has transformed countless lives. Her teachings transcend the mere use of herbs for ailments; they embody a philosophy of living in harmony with nature.

Barbara's teachings have not only influenced my personal health journey but have also shaped my approach to writing this book. Her holistic view of health, emphasizing the interconnectedness of physical, mental, and spiritual well-being, forms the foundation upon which the chapters of this book are built. Her belief in the body's inherent wisdom and its capacity to heal itself when supported by natural remedies is a message that I hope to convey through these pages.

A Journey Through Herbal Healing

As we traverse the chapters of this book, we will explore various facets of herbal healing. Each chapter is crafted to provide a comprehensive understanding of how herbal remedies can be integrated into our daily lives for better health and wellness.

The use of herbs for healing is an ancient practice, one that has stood the test of time. This book aims to bring that ancient wisdom into the context of our modern lives. It is about rediscovering the simplicity and efficacy of traditional remedies and understanding how they can be adapted to address the health challenges we face today.

The Role of Nature in Healing

In our fast-paced, technology-driven world, we often find ourselves disconnected from the natural environment. This disconnection can manifest in various forms of physical and mental health issues. By reconnecting with nature, not only do we find solace and peace, but we also tap into a powerful source of healing.

This book encourages you to view nature not just as a resource for ingredients but as a partner in healing. The plants, herbs, and natural elements around us are not mere commodities; they are part of a larger ecosystem to which we belong and with which we can interact to promote health and harmony.

The Importance of a Personalized Approach

Just as each plant has its unique properties and uses, each individual has unique health needs and conditions. This book aims to provide you with the knowledge and tools to understand how to select and use herbal remedies in a way that is most beneficial for your personal health.

In addition, the book addresses the importance of considering various factors such as lifestyle, diet, and emotional well-being when using herbal remedies. It's not just about treating symptoms; it's about addressing the root causes of health issues and fostering an overall state of well-being.

A Call to Embrace Holistic Well-Being

" Over 350 Barbara O'Neill Inspired Herbal Healing Home Remedies & Natural Medicine." is more than a guide to herbal remedies; it is a call to embrace a more holistic view of health. It's a call to take a step back from the often stressful modern life and find balance and health through nature's wisdom.

Whether you are new to the world of herbal medicine or have been exploring it for years, there is something in these pages for everyone. It is my hope that you will not only gain a deeper understanding of herbal remedies but also develop a greater appreciation for the intricate connection between our health and the natural world.

This book is an invitation to embark on a transformative journey, a journey that promises not just physical healing but also a deeper connection with the natural world and a more harmonious way of living.

I warmly invite you to turn the page and begin this enriching journey with me. Let us explore the world of herbal healing together, inspired by the timeless teachings of Barbara O'Neill and the countless healing stories of nature itself.

Important information! Why Our Book Does Not Include colored Herb Photos!

Consideration for Cost and Accessibility:

In our commitment to keeping the book affordable, we consciously decided against including color herb photos. This decision directly impacts and lowers the printing costs, making the book more accessible to a broader range of readers. Our priority is to provide comprehensive herbal knowledge at a reasonable price.

Emphasizing the Role of Visual Aids:

Understanding the importance of visual identification in herbal studies, especially for newcomers and in recipe preparation, we recommend for detailed herb images.

https://myplantin.com/plant-identifier/herb

This online resource complements our book perfectly, enabling accurate herb identification and enhancing your herbal learning experience.

CHAPTER 1: FOUNDATIONS OF HERBAL MEDICINE

This chapter, dedicated to the foundations of herbal medicine, is not merely an introduction to various herbs and their properties; it is a gateway to understanding the profound relationship between humans and the healing powers of the natural world. Herbal medicine, with its ancient roots and modern relevance, offers a unique perspective on health and wellness, emphasizing a harmonious balance between our bodies and the natural environment.

The Historical Context of Herbal Medicine

Herbal medicine is as ancient as humanity itself. From the dawn of civilization, humans have looked to plants and herbs for healing. This traditional knowledge, passed down through generations, forms the bedrock of many contemporary herbal practices. It is a rich tapestry of wisdom, encompassing a deep understanding of the natural properties of plants and their impact on the human body.

This historical perspective is crucial to appreciate fully the value of herbal medicine in our modern context. It provides a lens through which we can view herbal medicine not as a collection of remedies but as a holistic approach to health that has stood the test of time. This historical understanding also highlights the importance of preserving and respecting this ancient knowledge, ensuring its survival and relevance for future generations.

Understanding the Principles of Herbal Medicine

Herbal medicine is grounded in several core principles that guide its practice. Firstly, it is based on the understanding that every plant possesses unique properties that can be harnessed for healing purposes. These properties, ranging from the physical to the energetic, interact with the human body in complex ways.

Another fundamental principle is the holistic nature of herbal medicine. Unlike conventional medicine, which often focuses on treating specific symptoms, herbal medicine looks at the individual as a whole. This holistic approach takes into account not only physical symptoms but also emotional, mental, and spiritual well-being.

Additionally, herbal medicine is inherently personalized. It recognizes that each individual has unique health needs and responds differently to various herbs and treatments. This personalized approach is a key differentiator of herbal medicine, allowing for treatments that are tailored to the individual's specific conditions and constitution.

The Role of Herbs in Human Health

Herbs play a multifaceted role in human health. They are not only used for treating illnesses but also for preventing disease, maintaining wellness, and enhancing physical, mental, and emotional well-being. Herbs can be powerful allies in managing chronic conditions, supporting the body's natural healing processes, and promoting overall health and longevity.

To fully appreciate the role of herbs, one must understand their properties and how they interact with the human body. Each herb contains a unique combination of active compounds that impart specific therapeutic effects. These compounds can work synergistically, enhancing each other's effects, or they can be used individually to target specific health concerns.

The Art and Science of Herbal Medicine

Herbal medicine is both an art and a science. As a science, it requires a deep understanding of botany, chemistry, and human physiology. It involves studying the active constituents of plants, understanding their mechanisms of action, and researching their effects on the human body.

As an art, herbal medicine involves more than just knowledge of herbs and their properties; it requires intuition, wisdom, and a deep connection with the natural world. It involves understanding the subtle nuances of herbal remedies, knowing how to combine herbs synergistically, and tailoring treatments to the unique needs of each individual.

Cultivating a Relationship with Plants

A key aspect of herbal medicine is cultivating a relationship with plants. This involves more than just using plants for their medicinal properties; it involves developing a deep respect and reverence for them. It's about understanding that plants are living beings with their own energies and spirits, and learning to communicate with them.

This relationship with plants is central to the practice of herbal medicine. It involves spending time in nature, observing plants in their natural habitats, and learning to listen to what they have to teach us. This connection with plants enriches the practice of herbal medicine, making it a deeply fulfilling and transformative experience.

Herbal Medicine in the Modern World

In our modern world, where technology and pharmaceuticals dominate the healthcare landscape, herbal medicine offers a refreshing and vital alternative. It provides a way to reconnect with the natural world, to take control of our health, and to treat our bodies with the respect and care they deserve.

However, integrating herbal medicine into our modern lives requires a thoughtful and informed approach. It involves learning to discern credible information from misinformation, understanding the limitations and risks of herbal remedies, and knowing when to seek professional guidance.

EXPLORING HERBAL HEALING PRINCIPLES

In this exploration of the principles of herbal healing, we immerse ourselves into a world where nature is the healer and we, its willing apprentices. O'Neill's teachings provide a comprehensive framework for understanding and applying the ancient wisdom of herbal medicine in our contemporary lives.

The Holistic Approach

This perspective views the human being not as a collection of separate parts to be treated in isolation but as an integrated whole. In this view, physical ailments are often manifestations of imbalances that could be emotional, spiritual, or environmental in nature. Herbal healing, therefore, is not just about addressing the physical symptoms of a condition but about nurturing the entire being; body, mind, and spirit.

The approach also underscores the importance of prevention over cure. O'Neill teaches that maintaining health is not merely about reacting to illness but about creating a lifestyle that supports overall well-being. This encompasses a balanced diet, regular physical activity, mental and emotional wellness practices, and a harmonious relationship with our environment.

The Synergy of Herbs

O'Neill's teachings emphasize the synergy of herbs, the idea that herbs can work together in harmony to produce a more effective healing response than when used individually. This principle is rooted in the understanding that the compounds in herbs can complement and enhance each other's therapeutic effects. The art of creating herbal blends is a key aspect of her teachings, requiring a deep understanding of each herb's properties and how they interact with one another.

In line with this principle, O'Neill encourages practitioners to approach herbal blending with both scientific knowledge and intuitive understanding. This involves not only knowing the active constituents of herbs and their medicinal properties but also understanding the energetic qualities of herbs and how they can harmonize to address the specific needs of an individual.

Understanding the Energetics of Herbs

A unique aspect of O'Neill's approach to herbal healing is the emphasis on the energetics of herbs. This concept goes beyond the biochemical properties of plants to include their energetic qualities, such as warming, cooling, drying, and moistening. These qualities are considered in relation to the individual's constitution and the nature of their condition.

For instance, a person with a naturally warm and dry constitution experiencing inflammation (a hot and often dry condition) may benefit from herbs with cooling and moistening properties. This understanding of energetics allows for a more nuanced and personalized approach to herbal treatment.

The Connection with Nature

One of the most profound aspects of O'Neill's teachings is the deep connection with nature. She advocates for a relationship with the natural world that is based on respect, reverence, and reciprocity. This connection is not just about using nature's resources for our benefit but about understanding our place within the natural ecosystem and our responsibility to care for it.

O'Neill encourages practitioners and students of herbal medicine to spend time in nature, observing and learning from the plants. This immersive experience is seen as essential for developing a deep, intuitive understanding of herbal medicine.

The Empowerment of Self-Care

O'Neill's teachings centers on the empowerment of individuals in their health journey. She advocates for self-care and personal responsibility in health and wellness. This involves educating oneself about the principles of herbal medicine, understanding one's own body and its signals, and being proactive in maintaining health.

This empowerment is also about breaking free from the dependency on conventional medical systems and reclaiming the innate power of our bodies to heal. O'Neill teaches that with the right support, our bodies have an incredible capacity for self-healing and that herbs can be powerful allies in this process.

The Integration of Diet and Lifestyle

O'Neill's teachings integrate the use of herbs with dietary and lifestyle modifications. She emphasizes that herbs are most effective when used as part of a holistic approach to health that includes nutritious food, adequate rest, stress management, and regular physical activity.

In her view, diet is not just about nutrition; it's about nourishing the body and soul. It involves choosing foods that are natural, whole, and in alignment with our individual needs. Similarly, lifestyle choices are seen as important to maintaining health and preventing disease. This includes practices like mindfulness, meditation, and spending time in nature, all of which support overall well-being.

DIFFERENT HERBS AND THEIR HEALING PROPERTIES

Embarking on the exploration of various herbs and their healing properties opens us to a world where each leaf, root, and flower holds a story of healing and balance. This is the heart of herbal medicine, exploring the unique characteristics and uses of different herbs. These plants, revered by O'Neill for their medicinal properties, offer a natural pharmacy that can support our health in myriad ways.

The Healing Spectrum of Herbs

Each herb in nature's vast pharmacopeia brings its unique healing properties. O'Neill's teachings shed light on how these properties can be harnessed to address a wide range of health concerns, from the common cold to more complex chronic conditions. Understanding these properties requires not only an awareness of the active constituents of these herbs but also an appreciation for their roles in traditional and contemporary healing practices.

Adaptogenic Herbs for Stress and Balance

Adaptogens, a unique class of herbs, play a pivotal role in O'Neill's herbal repertoire. These herbs, including Ashwagandha, Rhodiola, and Holy basil, are known for their ability to help the body adapt to stress and restore balance. They work at a molecular level to moderate the stress response, enhancing resilience to physical, emotional, and environmental stressors.

Ashwagandha, for instance, has been revered for centuries in Ayurvedic medicine for its restorative and rejuvenating properties. It's known for its ability to support adrenal health, helping to mitigate the effects of stress and fatigue.

Herbs for Digestive Health

Digestive health is another area where O'Neill emphasizes the use of herbs. Herbs like Peppermint, Ginger, and Fennel are celebrated for their ability to soothe digestive discomfort, enhance nutrient absorption, and support gut health.

Peppermint, with its calming and antispasmodic properties, is particularly beneficial in relieving symptoms of indigestion and irritable bowel syndrome. Ginger, known for its warming and anti-inflammatory properties, can alleviate nausea and support healthy digestion.

Herbs for Immune Support

In the realm of immune support, O'Neill highlights the importance of herbs like Echinacea, Elderberry, and Astragalus. These herbs are renowned for their ability to bolster the body's defense mechanisms and enhance overall immunity.

Echinacea, for instance, is widely used for its immune-boosting properties, particularly in the prevention and treatment of colds and flu. Elderberry, rich in antioxidants, has a long history of use in supporting respiratory health.

Herbs for Cardiovascular Health

Cardiovascular health is also a key focus in these teachings. Herbs such as Hawthorn, Garlic, and Ginkgo biloba have been identified for their roles in supporting heart health and circulation. Hawthorn, for example, is known for its cardiotonic properties, improving heart function and promoting healthy circulation.

Herbal Nervines for Mental Well-being

O'Neill also places significance on herbs that support mental and emotional well-being, known as nervines. These include herbs like Lemon Balm, Lavender, and St. John's Wort. Lemon Balm, with its soothing properties, is used to alleviate anxiety and promote calmness. Lavender, renowned for its relaxing aroma, is widely used for stress relief and sleep support.

Herbs for Women's and Men's Health

These teachings also explore herbs specifically beneficial for women's and men's health. For women, herbs like Chaste tree (Vitex), Red raspberry Leaf, and Black Cohosh have been recognized for their efficacy in balancing hormones and addressing menstrual and menopausal issues.

In men's health, herbs such as Saw palmetto and Nettle Root are noted for their supportive role in prostate health and hormonal balance.

Culinary Herbs with Medicinal Properties

The healing power of herbs is not limited to those typically classified as medicinal; many culinary herbs also possess significant health benefits. Herbs like Turmeric, Cinnamon, and Rosemary, commonly used in cooking, are also powerful healers. Turmeric, with its active compound curcumin, is known for its potent anti-inflammatory and antioxidant properties.

The exploration of different herbs and their healing properties is a testament to the diversity and richness of nature's healing capabilities. These herbs, each with its unique profile of benefits, offer a comprehensive approach to health and wellness. They remind us of the interconnectedness of our health with the natural world and the immense potential that lies in understanding and utilizing these natural gifts responsibly and effectively. In the next section, we will further our research by examining the safe gathering and preparation techniques for these medicinal herbs, ensuring their benefits are harnessed to their fullest potential.

SAFE GATHERING AND PREPARATION TECHNIQUES

The art of herbal medicine extends far beyond the mere identification of herbs and their properties. It encompasses a deep understanding of how to safely gather and prepare these natural gifts. This subchapter digs into the practices essential for ensuring the potency and safety of herbal remedies. These practices are not only crucial for maximizing the healing benefits of herbs but also embody a deeper respect for nature and its resources.

The Ethics of Herbal Gathering

Before going into the technicalities of gathering herbs, it is crucial to understand the ethics that guide these practices. Ethical gathering is rooted in a profound respect for nature and its ecosystems. It involves taking only what is needed, ensuring that the harvesting of herbs does not deplete natural populations or disturb their natural habitat. This respect extends to seeking permission from landowners and recognizing the cultural significance of certain plants to indigenous communities.

O'Neill outlines the importance of sustainable gathering practices. This includes understanding the life cycle of plants, gathering at the appropriate time in the season to ensure regeneration, and being mindful of the impact of harvesting on the local ecosystem. For example, when gathering roots, one should only take a portion of the root system, leaving enough to allow the plant to recover and continue its growth cycle.

Identification and Quality

Accurate identification of herbs is a fundamental aspect of safe herbal gathering. Misidentification can lead to the use of the wrong herb, potentially causing harm. O'Neill advises the use of reliable field guides and, if possible, learning from experienced herbalists.

Assessing the quality of herbs is equally important. This involves examining the plants for signs of health and vitality. Healthy plants are more likely to have a higher concentration of beneficial compounds. Factors such as color, aroma, and texture can provide clues to the quality of the herb. For instance, vibrant colors and strong, fresh scents are often indicators of good quality.

Harvesting Techniques

Proper harvesting techniques are essential for preserving the integrity and medicinal properties of herbs. Different parts of the plant; leaves, flowers, roots, seeds, require different harvesting techniques. O'Neill teaches that leaves and flowers should be harvested when the plant is in its peak flowering stage, as this is when the concentration of active constituents is highest.

When harvesting roots, it is typically done in the fall when the plant's energy has moved back into the root system. Seeds are collected when they are fully mature and have begun to dry on the plant. The techniques of harvesting also include gentle handling to prevent bruising and damage to the plant tissues.

Drying and Storage

Once harvested, the proper drying and storage of herbs are crucial for maintaining their medicinal qualities. O'Neill's guidelines suggest that herbs should be dried quickly to prevent the growth of mold and the degradation of active compounds. Methods of drying include air drying, using a dehydrator, or in some cases, oven drying at a low temperature.

The storage of dried herbs is equally important. Herbs should be stored in airtight containers away from direct sunlight and moisture. Glass jars with tight-fitting lids are ideal for this purpose. Properly dried and stored herbs can retain their potency for up to a year.

Preparation Techniques

The preparation of herbal remedies is an art that requires both knowledge and intuition. O'Neill's teachings cover various preparation methods, including infusions, decoctions, tinctures, and salves.

Infusions, similar to making tea, involve pouring boiling water over the herb and allowing it to steep. This method is suitable for delicate parts of the plant, such as leaves and flowers. Decoctions involve simmering tougher parts, like roots and bark, in water to extract their medicinal properties.

Salves and ointments, made by infusing herbs in oils and then blending with waxes, are used for topical applications. These preparations are beneficial for skin conditions and as healing balms.

Safety Considerations in Preparation

Safety in the preparation of herbal remedies is paramount. This includes understanding the correct dosages and recognizing that some herbs can have potent effects or interact with medications. O'Neill emphasizes the importance of starting with small doses and observing the body's response.

Understanding contraindications is also crucial. Some herbs should not be used during pregnancy or by individuals with certain health conditions. Accurate knowledge and careful consideration of these factors are essential in the safe preparation of herbal remedies.

The gathering and preparation of herbs are practices that require respect, knowledge, and a deep connection with the natural world. These practices are not just about creating remedies but about fostering a relationship with nature that is ethical, sustainable, and mindful.

Chapter 2: Herbal Safety and Contraindications

In herbal medicine, as in all forms of healing, the first principle is to do no harm. This chapter teaches the critical aspects of herbal safety and contraindications, an area often overshadowed by the allure of herbal remedies' benefits. Understanding these facets is essential for anyone venturing into the world of herbal medicine, whether as a practitioner, student, or consumer.

The Imperative of Safety in Herbal Medicine

The rising popularity of herbal remedies brings with it the need for a heightened awareness of their safe use. While herbs are natural, it is a misconception that they are inherently safe. Like any therapeutic intervention, they come with their own set of risks and benefits. Safety in herbal medicine involves understanding these risks, knowing how to minimize them, and recognizing when and how to use these remedies effectively.

Understanding Herbal Actions and Constituents

The safety of herbal remedies is deeply tied to their actions and constituents. Herbs contain a variety of active compounds, each with specific effects on the body. For instance, some herbs may have a sedative effect, while others may stimulate the nervous system. Understanding these actions is crucial in predicting how an herb might interact with the body, other herbs, or pharmaceutical medications.

The constituents of herbs, such as alkaloids, glycosides, and flavonoids, also play a significant role in their safety profile. These chemical compounds can have potent physiological effects, beneficial in some contexts and potentially harmful in others. An in-depth understanding of these constituents forms the basis for recognizing contraindications and potential adverse effects.

Identifying and Managing Allergic Reactions

One of the primary safety concerns in herbal medicine is the risk of allergic reactions. Just as with foods and other substances, individuals can have allergic reactions to certain herbs. These reactions can range from mild, such as rashes or itching, to severe, such as anaphylaxis. Identifying and managing these reactions is a vital aspect of safe herbal practice. This involves careful screening for allergies, monitoring for signs of reaction during herbal treatment, and having protocols in place to address any adverse reactions.

Contraindications and Special Populations

Certain populations require special consideration when it comes to herbal treatments. These include pregnant and breastfeeding women, children, the elderly, and individuals with specific health conditions, such as liver or kidney disease. For these groups, certain herbs may be contraindicated, or specific dosages may need to be adjusted. Understanding these contraindications is crucial to prevent harm and ensure the safe use of herbal remedies.

Interactions with Pharmaceuticals

As herbal medicine often complements conventional treatments, understanding the potential interactions between herbs and pharmaceutical medications is crucial. Some herbs can potentiate or diminish the effects of certain drugs, leading to increased side effects or reduced therapeutic efficacy. This area of study requires not only a deep knowledge of herbal constituents but also an understanding of pharmacodynamics and pharmacokinetics.

The Importance of Dosage and Formulation

Dosage and formulation are key factors in the safety of herbal medicine. The therapeutic dose of an herb can vary widely depending on the individual, the condition being treated, and the specific herb or herbs being used. Overdosing can lead to adverse effects, while underdosing may render the treatment ineffective.

The formulation of herbal remedies, including the method of preparation and the part of the plant used, also significantly impacts their safety and effectiveness. For instance, certain herbs are safe and beneficial in a tea form but can be harmful if concentrated into an extract.

Responsible Sourcing and Quality Control

The safety of herbal remedies is not only determined by their inherent properties and how they are used but also by the quality of the herbs themselves. Responsible sourcing and quality control are essential to ensure that herbs are free from contaminants such as pesticides, heavy metals, and adulterants. This includes understanding the origin of herbs, the conditions under which they were grown and harvested, and the processes used in their drying and storage.

The Role of Education and Awareness

A key theme in O'Neill's teachings is the importance of education and awareness in the safe use of herbal remedies. This involves not only educating practitioners and students but also consumers who choose to use these remedies. Increasing awareness about the potential risks, contraindications, and safe practices can empower individuals to make informed decisions about their use of herbal medicine.

This chapter on herbal safety and contraindications is a foundational element of responsible herbal practice. It stresses the need for a balanced approach to herbal medicine, one that respects its power to heal and acknowledges its potential risks. By deepening our understanding of these aspects, we can use herbal remedies not only effectively but safely, ensuring that the practice of herbal medicine continues to be a source of healing and wellbeing.

REFLECTIVE SEGMENT ON UNDERSTANDING HERBAL SAFETY

As we practice use of herbal medicine, it becomes imperative to pause and reflect on the concept of herbal safety. This reflective segment aims to deepen our understanding of what it truly means to use herbs safely. It's not merely about following guidelines or adhering to dosages; it's about cultivating a mindset and approach that respects the power of these natural entities and recognizes the intricate ways in which they interact with our bodies and our environment.

The Complexity of Herbal Interactions

The world of herbal medicine is vast and complex. Herbs, with their myriad of constituents, can interact with our bodies in multifaceted ways. These interactions are not always straightforward and can vary depending on individual factors such as age, genetics, overall health, and concurrent use of medications or other herbs.

This complexity demands a thoughtful and cautious approach to using herbs. It requires us to be diligent in our research and humble in our assertions. Recognizing that our understanding of herbs and their interactions is continually evolving, we must remain open to new information and be willing to adjust our practices accordingly.

The Individuality of Herbal Response

Each person's response to a particular herb can be unique. Factors like metabolic rate, digestive health, and even emotional state can influence how an individual responds to a herbal remedy. This individuality necessitates a personalized approach to herbal medicine, where remedies are tailored to the specific needs and conditions of the individual.

Reflecting on this individuality also highlights the importance of close observation and communication. Practitioners must be attentive to the responses of their clients and be prepared to modify treatments as necessary. Similarly, individuals using herbs must be attuned to their bodies and communicate any unexpected reactions to their healthcare providers.

The Responsibility of Accurate Information

In an age where information is readily available but not always accurate, the responsibility of disseminating and obtaining correct information about herbal safety is paramount. Misinformation can lead to misuse of herbs, resulting in ineffective treatment or, worse, harm. This responsibility falls on practitioners, educators, and consumers alike.

For practitioners and educators, this means ensuring that the information they share is based on credible sources and is presented in a manner that is understandable and accessible to their audience. For consumers, it involves seeking out reliable information and being discerning about the sources they trust.

The Role of Education in Herbal Safety

Education plays a critical role in ensuring the safe use of herbs. This education should extend beyond the basic knowledge of herbs and their uses. It should encompass an understanding of how to evaluate the quality of herbal products, how to recognize signs of quality and contamination, and how to store and handle herbs properly to maintain their potency and safety.

Moreover, education in herbal safety should also include learning how to recognize and respond to adverse reactions. This involves understanding the signs of allergic reactions, herb-drug interactions, and toxicity. It also includes knowing when to seek professional medical help.

The Ethics of Herbal Consumption

Reflecting on herbal safety also involves considering the ethical aspects of herbal consumption. This includes the sustainability of herbal sourcing, the impact of our consumption on the environment, and respect for the cultural origins of various herbal practices. As consumers and practitioners of herbal medicine, it's important to make choices that are not only safe for us as individuals but also for the larger community and the planet.

Practicing Mindfulness and Intuition

Mindfulness and intuition are invaluable tools in the practice of herbal safety. Being mindful means being fully present and aware during the preparation and use of herbal remedies. It involves paying attention to details, being conscious of the process, and being attuned to the response of the body.

Intuition, while often overlooked in the scientific discourse, plays a significant role in herbal medicine. It involves listening to the subtle cues of the body and the herbs, and trusting one's inner wisdom to guide the healing process. Developing this intuition requires time, experience, and a deep connection with both the self and the natural world.

Navigating the Challenges of Herbal Safety

Navigating the challenges of herbal safety requires a balance of knowledge, experience, and caution. It involves being proactive in learning and staying updated with the latest research while also being cautious in applying this knowledge. It requires being open to learning from mistakes and being willing to adapt and evolve.

Understanding herbal safety is a multifaceted and ongoing process. It involves a deep appreciation of the complexities of herbal interactions, the individuality of responses to herbs, the responsibility of providing and obtaining accurate information, and the importance of education.

IDENTIFYING POTENTIAL SIDE EFFECTS AND INTERACTIONS

In the field of herbal medicine, recognizing and understanding the potential side effects and interactions of herbs is as crucial as acknowledging their healing properties. This subchapter accentuates the vital aspect of identifying potential side effects and interactions associated with herbal remedies. This understanding is not just a precaution but a fundamental component of responsible herbal practice, ensuring that the path to healing remains safe and informed.

Comprehending the Scope of Side Effects

Herbal medicine is often marked by the allure of natural healing. However, it is essential to remember that 'natural' does not automatically imply 'without side effects.' Herbs, like any therapeutic agents, can cause adverse reactions in some individuals. These reactions can range from mild to severe and may manifest as allergies, digestive disturbances, headaches, or more significant complications depending on the individual and the herb in question.

Understanding the scope of these side effects involves more than just a cursory glance at a list of possible reactions. It requires a deep dive into the herb's pharmacology, understanding the mechanisms by which these effects occur.

Monitoring and Managing Side Effects

The proactive monitoring of side effects is a critical component of safe herbal practice. This involves being vigilant about observing any changes that occur after beginning an herbal regimen and being prepared to adjust or discontinue the use of the herb if necessary. It also includes educating individuals about the signs and symptoms to watch for and encouraging open communication about their experiences.

Managing side effects, when they do occur, requires much caution. Depending on the severity and nature of the reaction, this might involve reducing the dosage, changing the method of preparation, or discontinuing the herb altogether. In some cases, supportive treatments may be necessary to alleviate the side effects.

Herb-Drug Interactions: A Critical Consideration

In our modern healthcare landscape, where many individuals are on conventional medications, the potential for herb-drug interactions is a significant concern. These interactions can affect the metabolism of drugs, either increasing their potency and thereby enhancing their side effects or reducing their efficacy.

Navigating herb-drug interactions requires an understanding of pharmacokinetics and pharmacodynamics. It involves knowing how herbs can affect the absorption, distribution, metabolism, and excretion of drugs. O'Neill advocates for careful review and consideration of an individual's medication regimen before recommending or using herbal remedies.

The Importance of Comprehensive Health Assessment

A comprehensive health assessment is critical in identifying potential side effects and interactions. This assessment should include a detailed medical history, an understanding of the individual's current health status, and a thorough review of any medications or supplements they are taking.

This allows practitioners to make informed decisions about which herbs are appropriate and safe for each individual.

SPECIAL PRECAUTIONS FOR CONDITIONS AND MEDICATIONS

In the intricacy of herbal medicine, special precautions for certain conditions and medications form an essential thread. This aspect of herbal practice demands careful consideration and deep understanding. It involves acknowledging that while herbs offer immense healing potential, they must be used judiciously, especially in the presence of specific health conditions and medications.

Navigating Herbal Use in Chronic Conditions

When dealing with chronic conditions such as heart disease, diabetes, or kidney disorders, the use of herbal remedies requires careful consideration. O'Neill's teachings guide us to approach such scenarios with a blend of wisdom and caution. Herbs that may generally be safe for the average person can have different implications for someone with a chronic condition.

For example, in cardiovascular diseases, herbs that affect blood pressure or heart rate, like Hawthorn or Ginseng, must be used under professional guidance. Their interaction with heart medications or their impact on heart function demands careful monitoring.

In the context of diabetes, herbs that influence blood sugar levels, such as Gymnema or Fenugreek, require cautious use. Their potential to significantly lower blood sugar levels can be a concern, especially when used alongside conventional diabetes medications.

Herbal Use in Pregnancy and Lactation

The use of herbs during pregnancy and lactation is another area where O'Neill's teachings emphasize caution. Many herbs that are typically safe can have contraindications during pregnancy due to their potential to stimulate uterine contractions or affect hormone levels.

For example, herbs like Mugwort or Pennyroyal, while useful in certain contexts, are strongly contraindicated in pregnancy due to their potential to induce miscarriage. Similarly, during lactation, herbs that can be transferred through breast milk and impact the infant, such as Peppermint or Parsley, which can reduce milk supply, must be used with caution.

Age-Related Considerations in Herbal Medicine

O'Neill's approach to herbal safety also considers the age of the individual. Children and the elderly, for instance, have different physiological responses and sensitivities to herbs. In children, the liver and kidneys, responsible for metabolizing and excreting substances, are not fully developed. This factor necessitates lower dosages and the avoidance of certain potent herbs.

In the elderly, decreased liver and kidney function, along with the common presence of multiple medications, calls for a cautious approach. Herbs that may affect hydration levels or interact with medications commonly used by older adults need to be used judiciously.

Mental Health Conditions and Herbal Considerations

When it comes to mental health conditions, such as anxiety, depression, or insomnia, the use of herbs requires a nuanced understanding. While many herbs can support mental health, they can also interact with psychiatric medications.

Herbs like Valerian or Kava, used for their calming effects, may enhance the sedative effect of psychiatric drugs, leading to increased drowsiness or lethargy. Similarly, herbs with mood-enhancing properties should be used carefully in conjunction with antidepressants to avoid excessive serotonin levels, a condition known as serotonin syndrome.

The Complexity of Autoimmune Disorders

In autoimmune disorders, where the body's immune system attacks its tissues, the use of immunomodulating herbs needs careful consideration. Herbs that stimulate the immune system may exacerbate symptoms in autoimmune conditions.

Conversely, immunosuppressive herbs might offer relief but could also reduce the body's ability to fight infections.

The Impact of Herbs on Liver and Kidney Functions

For individuals with liver or kidney diseases, certain herbs can pose significant risks. Herbs metabolized through the liver or having hepatotoxic potential must be used with extreme caution in liver disorders. Similarly, herbs that are diuretics or have high mineral content can strain the kidneys in kidney diseases.

Following special precautions for specific conditions and medications is a cornerstone of safe and effective herbal practice. It involves a thorough understanding of the individual's health status, a deep knowledge of how herbs interact with various conditions and medications, and a commitment to continual learning and adaptation.

Important information! Why Our Book Does Not Include colored Herb Photos!

Consideration for Cost and Accessibility:

In our commitment to keeping the book affordable, we consciously decided against including color herb photos. This decision directly impacts and lowers the printing costs, making the book more accessible to a broader range of readers. Our priority is to provide comprehensive herbal knowledge at a reasonable price.

Emphasizing the Role of Visual Aids:

Understanding the importance of visual identification in herbal studies, especially for newcomers and in recipe preparation, we recommend for detailed herb images.

https://myplantin.com/plant-identifier/herb

This online resource complements our book perfectly, enabling accurate herb identification and enhancing your herbal learning experience.

CHAPTER 3: HERBAL REMEDIES FOR COMMON AILMENTS

Journeying through the world of herbal medicine, one of the most rewarding destinations is the discovery of remedies for common ailments. This chapter probes the heart of practical herbalism by exploring the use of herbal remedies to address everyday health issues. While modern medicine often seeks to treat symptoms through standardized treatments, herbal medicine offers a more personalized approach, harnessing the natural potency of plants to heal and restore balance.

The Philosophy of Treating Common Ailments with Herbs

The philosophy underpinning the use of herbal remedies for common ailments is grounded in the principles of holism and balance. It's rooted in the understanding that the body is a self-regulating system, capable of healing itself given the right support. Herbal remedies work in harmony with the body's natural processes, gently nudging it back to health, rather than overpowering it with aggressive treatments.

Herbal Approaches to Digestive Issues

Digestive issues such as indigestion, constipation, and diarrhea are common ailments where herbal remedies can be particularly effective. The gentle, yet powerful properties of herbs like ginger, peppermint, and chamomile can soothe the digestive tract, reduce inflammation, and promote regularity. Unlike many over-the-counter remedies that offer temporary relief, these herbs address the root causes of digestive discomfort.

Respiratory Conditions and Herbal Treatments

For respiratory conditions like the common cold, cough, and sinusitis, herbal medicine offers a wealth of remedies. Herbs such as echinacea, elderberry, and thyme possess properties that can boost the immune system, alleviate congestion, and soothe irritated respiratory passages. These herbs not only provide symptomatic relief but also assist the body's natural defense mechanisms in combating infections.

Herbal Solutions for Skin Ailments

Skin ailments, including eczema, acne, and psoriasis, can also be effectively managed with herbal remedies. Herbs such as calendula, Aloe vera, and Tea tree oil have healing, anti-inflammatory, and antimicrobial properties that can soothe the skin, reduce inflammation, and promote healing. These natural remedies offer a gentler alternative to harsh chemical treatments, nurturing the skin back to health.

Managing Stress and Anxiety with Herbs

Herbs offer invaluable support for managing stress and anxiety. Adaptogenic herbs like ashwagandha and Holy basil help the body adapt to stress, while nervine herbs like lemon balm and lavender provide a calming effect. These herbs work not just on the symptoms of stress and anxiety but on the overall resilience of the nervous system.

Herbal Remedies for Sleep Disturbances

Sleep disturbances, a common ailment in our fast-paced world, can also be effectively addressed with herbs. Herbal remedies such as valerian root, passionflower, and hops have sedative properties that can help improve the quality of sleep. These herbs offer a natural alternative to sleep medications, helping to induce a restful sleep without the risk of dependency.

Addressing Pain and Inflammation with Herbal Remedies

Herbs can be powerful allies in managing pain and inflammation. Anti-inflammatory herbs like turmeric, ginger, and Willow bark can be as effective as conventional anti-inflammatory drugs in some cases, without the associated side effects. These herbs can be used for a range of conditions, from arthritis and menstrual cramps to headaches and muscle pain.

The Role of Herbs in Women's and Men's Health

In women's health, herbs play a significant role in managing conditions like menstrual cramps, premenstrual syndrome, and menopausal symptoms. Herbs like Chaste tree, black cohosh, and Red raspberry leaf offer natural support for hormonal balance and relief from symptoms. In men's health, herbs like Saw palmetto and nettle root are used for prostate health and urinary issues, providing natural support for common men's health concerns.

Herbal remedies offer a treasure trove of healing for common ailments. Their power lies in their ability to work in harmony with the body's natural processes, offering relief and promoting healing without overwhelming the body's delicate balance.

DETAILED RECIPES FOR TREATING COMMON CONDITIONS INSPIRED BY O'NEILL'S REMEDIES

In the landscape of natural healing, the creation of herbal remedies is both an art and a science. This subchapter is dedicated to crafting detailed recipes for treating common conditions. These recipes are more than mere mixtures of herbs; they are carefully composed blends that harness the individual strengths of each herb to create a synergistic effect. We will explore a variety of conditions and the corresponding herbal remedies, emphasizing the practical application of O'Neill's teachings in everyday health management.

Recipe for Digestive Tea:
- Peppermint leaves: 1 teaspoon
- Ginger root (freshly grated): 1 teaspoon
- Fennel seeds: ½ teaspoon
- Boiling water: 1 cup

Steep the peppermint leaves, ginger root, and fennel seeds in boiling water for 10 minutes. Strain and drink the tea warm. This tea can be consumed after meals to aid digestion or when experiencing indigestion.

Recipe for Respiratory Syrup:
- Dried elderberries: ½ cup
- Echinacea root: ¼ cup
- Thyme leaves: ¼ cup
- Water: 3 cups
- Honey: 1 cup

Simmer elderberries, echinacea root, and thyme leaves in water for about 30 minutes. Strain the mixture, add Honey, and stir until dissolved. Store the syrup in a glass bottle in the refrigerator. Take 1 tablespoon every four hours during a cold.

Recipe for Skin Ailments
- Dried calendula flowers: ½ cup
- Aloe vera gel: 1 cup
- Beeswax: ¼ cup
- Olive oil: ½ cup

Infuse calendula flowers in olive oil over low heat for 2 hours. Strain the flowers and combine the infused oil with beeswax, melting them together. Once slightly cooled, mix in the Aloe vera gel. Pour into containers and allow to solidify. Apply to affected skin areas as needed.

Recipe for Calming Tea:
- Dried lemon balm: 1 teaspoon
- Dried lavender flowers: 1 teaspoon
- Dried chamomile flowers: 1 teaspoon
- Boiling water: 1 cup

Mix the herbs and steep in boiling water for 10 minutes. Strain and drink the tea warm, preferably in the evening or during times of stress.

Recipe for Sleep Aid Tincture:
- Dried valerian root: ¼ cup
- Dried passionflower: ¼ cup
- Dried hops: ¼ cup
- Apple cider vinegar (Barbara do not recommend using cider vinegar): 2 cups

Combine the valerian root, passionflower, and hops in a jar. Cover with Apple cider vinegar, ensuring the herbs are completely submerged. Seal the jar and store it in a cool, dark place for 4 to 6 weeks, shaking it daily. After steeping, strain the tincture and store it in amber dropper bottles. Use 20-30 drops in a little water before bedtime.

Recipe for Anti-Inflammatory Tea:
- Dried turmeric root: 1 teaspoon
- Dried ginger root: 1 teaspoon
- Dried Willow bark: ½ teaspoon
- Boiling water: 1 cup

Combine the turmeric, ginger, and Willow bark in a teapot. Pour boiling water over the herbs and steep for 15 minutes. Strain and drink the tea warm. It can be consumed up to twice daily for pain relief.

Recipe for Menstrual Relief Tincture:
- Dried Chaste tree berries: ¼ cup
- Dried black cohosh root: ¼ cup
- Dried Red raspberry leaf: ¼ cup
- Apple cider vinegar (Barbara do not recommend using cider vinegar): 2 cups

Combine the herbs in a jar and cover with vinegar. Seal the jar and let it sit for 4 to 6 weeks, shaking it daily. Strain and store the tincture in amber bottles. Use 20-30 drops in water, taken daily, especially during the second half of the menstrual cycle.

Recipe for Prostate Health Tea:
- Dried Saw palmetto berries: 1 teaspoon
- Dried nettle root: 1 teaspoon
- Boiling water: 1 cup

Steep the Saw palmetto berries and nettle root in boiling water for 10 minutes. Strain and consume the tea warm, ideally twice daily.

The creation of herbal medicine for common ailments, is a testament to the gentle yet profound power of nature in addressing everyday health challenges. These recipes provide practical, natural solutions, emphasizing the importance of understanding individual herbs and their synergistic effects.

In crafting and using these herbs, we also honor the traditions of herbalists who have come before us. We become part of a lineage of healers who have relied on the wisdom of nature to nurture health and healing. This connection to tradition enriches our modern lives, providing a sense of continuity and grounding in an ever-changing world.

These recipes are not just formulas to be followed; they are gateways to a deeper understanding of health and healing. They encourage us to explore, to experiment, and to find the unique combinations and preparations that work best for our individual needs.

In the following chapters, we will revisit many of these recipes and expand upon them in greater detail, so stay tuned for more insights and practical tips, also make sure to **visit the last chapter after the conclusion of the book** for a compilation of **over 300 Detailed Recipes for Treating Common Conditions Inspired by O'Neill's Remedies.**

INSTRUCTIONS FOR PREPARATION AND USAGE

Embarking on the use of herbal remedies involves more than just knowing which herbs to use for which ailments. It encompasses an understanding of the details involved in their preparation and usage. This subchapter focuses on the intricate processes of preparing and using herbal remedies. These processes are crucial for maximizing the efficacy and safety of the herbs, ensuring that their healing potential is fully realized.

The Art of Herbal Infusions

Herbal infusions are one of the simplest yet most effective ways to extract the healing properties of herbs. The process involves steeping herbs in hot water, which allows their medicinal compounds to be released. O'Neill emphasizes the importance of temperature and time in this process. For instance, delicate herbs like chamomile and lavender should be infused in just-boiled water for about 5 to 10 minutes to prevent the loss of their volatile oils. In contrast, more robust herbs like nettle or Red raspberry leaf require longer steeping times, typically around 15 to 20 minutes, to fully extract their beneficial properties.

Decoctions for Tougher Plant Materials

Decoctions are ideal for extracting the medicinal properties from tougher plant materials like roots, barks, and seeds. The process involves simmering these parts in water for an extended period, usually ranging from 20 minutes to an hour, depending on the hardness of the material. O'Neill advises that the water should initially be brought to a boil and then reduced to a simmer. This slow process allows for the deep extraction of medicinal compounds. For example, a decoction of burdock root, known for its blood-purifying properties, should be simmered for at least 30 minutes to ensure the extraction of its active constituents.

Topical Applications: Salves and Poultices

For external ailments, O'Neill often recommends the use of salves and poultices. Salves are made by infusing herbs in oils and then blending them with beeswax to create a thick, spreadable ointment. The choice of herbs depends on the condition being treated. For instance, a calendula salve can be used for skin irritations and minor wounds. Poultices involve applying herbs directly to the skin or using a soft cloth soaked in a herbal infusion or decoction. They are particularly useful for localized issues like inflammation or muscle pain.

Herbal Baths and Washes

Herbal baths and washes are another aspect of O'Neill's method, offering a soothing and therapeutic way to use herbs.

A herbal bath involves adding a strong infusion or decoction of herbs to bathwater, providing a relaxing and healing experience. Herbal washes, on the other hand, are used to cleanse or treat specific areas of the body. For example, an eye wash made from eyebright or chamomile can help relieve eye irritation or inflammation.

Customizing Herbal Remedies

Customization is a hallmark of O'Neill's approach to herbal preparation and usage. She encourages practitioners and individuals to tailor remedies to the specific needs and responses of each person. This means not only adjusting dosages but also combining herbs in unique ways to enhance their therapeutic effects. For instance, a sleep aid tincture might be customized with a blend of valerian, hops, and lavender for one individual, while another might benefit more from a combination of chamomile, passionflower, and lemon balm.

The Importance of Record-Keeping

O'Neill also emphasizes the importance of meticulous record-keeping when preparing and using herbal remedies. Documenting the herbs used, their sources, the methods of preparation, dosages, and the individual's responses, helps in refining treatments and tracking progress over time. This practice is particularly crucial for those who prepare their herbal remedies or for practitioners managing multiple clients.

Mindfulness in Herbal Preparation and Usage

Mindfulness in the preparation and usage of herbal remedies is a key aspect of O'Neill's teachings. This involves being fully present during the process of preparing the remedy, paying close attention to the colors, textures, and scents of the herbs, and being aware of their effects on the body. Such mindfulness enhances the therapeutic experience and deepens the individual's connection to the healing process.

Respecting the Limits of Herbal Medicine

While advocating for the benefits of herbal remedies, O'Neill also stresses the importance of understanding and respecting their limits. This includes recognizing when a condition requires conventional medical intervention and avoiding the use of herbs as a substitute for necessary medical care. Her approach is one of complementary use, where herbal remedies support and enhance overall health and wellbeing, rather than replace conventional treatments.

Continued Learning and Adaptation

Finally, this approach to herbal preparation and usage is characterized by a commitment to continued learning and adaptation. The field of herbal medicine is ever-evolving, with ongoing research shedding new light on the properties and uses of herbs. Staying informed about the latest developments, being open to new insights, and adapting practices accordingly are essential for ensuring the safe and effective use of herbal remedies.

DOSAGE AND FREQUENCY TIPS RECOMMENDED BY O'NEILL

Navigating the world of herbal medicine involves a keen understanding of the appropriate dosage and frequency of herbal medicines. This subchapter digs into the detailed art of determining how much and how often one should consume herbal preparations. These recommendations are not arbitrary; they are derived from a deep understanding of the herbs' properties, the individual's unique constitution, and the specific condition being treated.

The Principle of Start Low, Go Slow

One of the fundamental principles in determining dosage and frequency in herbal medicine, is to start with low doses and gradually increase as needed. This approach allows the body to adjust to the herb and helps in identifying the minimal effective dose; the lowest amount needed to achieve the desired therapeutic effect. This principle is particularly important when working with potent herbs or when treating sensitive individuals, such as children or the elderly.

Dosage Considerations

The determination of the correct dosage depends on several factors, including the age, weight, and health status of the individual, as well as the nature of the herb and the condition being treated. For example, children and elderly individuals generally require smaller doses than healthy adults due to differences in metabolism and body composition.

Additionally, the potency of the herb plays a significant role in dosage determination. Strongly acting herbs, such as those with sedative or laxative properties, typically require smaller doses, while milder herbs may be used in larger quantities.

Frequency of Herbal Intake

The frequency of taking an herbal remedy is as important as the dosage. This factor is influenced by the herb's duration of action and the nature of the condition being treated. Acute conditions, like a cold or an upset stomach, may require more frequent dosing of certain herbs to maintain steady therapeutic levels in the body. Chronic conditions, on the other hand, might benefit from less frequent dosing over a longer period.

O'Neill advises attention to the body's responses when determining frequency. Some individuals may experience relief with less frequent doses, while others may require more regular intake to achieve the desired effects.

Herb-Specific Dosage Guidelines

O'Neill's approach includes specific dosage guidelines for different herbs, recognizing that each herb has its unique profile. For instance, herbs like echinacea, used for immune support, may be taken in higher doses at the onset of symptoms and then reduced as the condition improves. Conversely, tonifying herbs like ashwagandha may be taken in consistent doses over an extended period to build and maintain energy levels.

Adjusting Dosage and Frequency Over Time

An important aspect of O'Neill's methodology is the adjustment of dosage and frequency over time. As the individual's condition changes, so too should the herbal treatment plan. This might mean reducing the dose as symptoms improve or increase it if the desired effect is not achieved.

Additionally, the duration of herbal treatment is a critical consideration. Some herbal remedies are meant for short-term use, while others can be taken safely over longer periods. Understanding the appropriate duration of treatment is essential to prevent potential side effects or tolerance to the herb's effects.

The Role of Personalization in Dosage and Frequency

Personalization is key in O'Neill's approach to dosage and frequency. She emphasizes that herbal medicine is not a one-size-fits-all solution. What works for one individual may not be effective for another, even with the same condition. This variability necessitates a tailored approach, considering the individual's unique physiological makeup, lifestyle, and specific health needs.

Educating on the Importance of Adherence

O'Neill stresses the importance of educating individuals on the significance of adherence to the prescribed dosage and frequency. Adherence ensures the effectiveness of the treatment and reduces the risk of adverse effects. For instance, sporadic intake of an herbal remedy meant to be taken regularly can lead to suboptimal results, while overuse can cause potential harm.

Monitoring and Feedback

Continuous monitoring and feedback are crucial components in adjusting dosage and frequency. O'Neill advises individuals to observe their responses to the herbal treatment closely and communicate any changes or concerns. This feedback loop allows for timely adjustments and ensures that the treatment remains aligned with the individual's evolving health status.

Understanding Herbal Forms and Their Dosages

Different forms of herbal preparations, such as teas, tinctures, capsules, and topicals, require different dosing considerations. O'Neill provides guidance on adjusting dosages based on the form of the herb being used. For example, tinctures are more concentrated than teas and thus require smaller dosages. Understanding these differences is essential for effective and safe herbal treatment.

The Importance of Consistency

Consistency in taking herbal remedies, as per the recommended dosage and frequency, is vital for achieving the desired therapeutic outcomes. O'Neill emphasizes the role of routine in herbal treatment, encouraging individuals to integrate the intake of herbal remedies into their daily schedules in a way that promotes consistent use.

Cautions and Contraindications

O'Neill's teachings also include cautions regarding the contraindications of certain herbs based on dosage and frequency. For instance, herbs that can impact hormonal balance, such as licorice or dong quai, must be used judiciously, considering factors like hormonal status and concurrent use of hormone-related medications.

The Role of Professional Guidance

In O'Neill's practice, the role of professional guidance in determining dosage and frequency is highly valued. Consulting with a knowledgeable herbalist or healthcare provider ensures that the herbal treatment plan is safe, effective, and tailored to the individual's specific needs. This professional input is particularly crucial when dealing with complex health conditions or when using potent herbs.

Balancing Tradition with Modern Understanding

In her approach, O'Neill balances traditional herbal wisdom with modern scientific understanding. This balance is reflected in her recommendations for dosage and frequency, which are grounded in historical use and supported by contemporary research where available.

The determination of appropriate dosage and frequency in herbal medicine is a dynamic and individualized process. It requires a deep understanding of herbal properties, personal health factors, and various herbal forms.

CHAPTER 4: SPECIALIZED HERBAL TREATMENTS

Herbal medicine extends far beyond general wellness and common ailments. It goes into a deeper, more intricate territory of specialized treatments, where herbs are used not just for their general healing properties but are carefully chosen and combined to address specific health conditions. This chapter explores the art and science of specialized herbal treatments. It is a walk into the heart of therapeutic herbalism, where the true power of herbs is harnessed to provide relief and healing for a range of specific health challenges.

The Essence of Specialized Herbalism

Specialized herbal treatments are based on the premise that each herb possesses unique properties that can be strategically used to target specific health issues. This approach is akin to a master craftsman selecting the perfect tools for a delicate job. It requires an in-depth understanding of each herb's pharmacological profile, including its active constituents, therapeutic actions, and potential side effects and interactions.

This level of understanding allows herbalists to create formulations that are not only effective in alleviating symptoms but also in addressing the underlying causes of health conditions. It is an approach that values the complexity of human health and respects the intricate ways in which our bodies interact with herbal constituents.

A Holistic Approach to Specific Conditions

Herbs are chosen not only for their direct impact on a particular condition but also for their ability to support the body's overall health and balance. This perspective recognizes that the body is an interconnected system, where treating one part affects the whole.

For example, in treating a condition like arthritis, the herbal treatment plan may include anti-inflammatory herbs to reduce joint pain and swelling, but it may also include herbs to support the liver and kidneys, which are vital in managing the body's inflammatory response and in processing the by-products of inflammation.

The Art of Herbal Synergy

A key concept in specialized herbal treatments is synergy, where the combined effect of herbs used together is greater than the sum of their individual effects. This synergy is not a matter of chance; it is carefully crafted based on the understanding of how different herbs interact and enhance each other's properties.

Creating a synergistic herbal formula requires a deep understanding of the nuances of herbal actions and an intuitive sense of how herbs will work together. It is an art form that is honed through experience, study, and a deep connection with the plant world.

Addressing Complex Health Issues

Specialized herbal treatments are particularly valuable in addressing complex health issues that do not respond well to conventional treatments or that require a more nuanced approach. Conditions such as chronic fatigue syndrome, autoimmune disorders, and hormonal imbalances are examples where specialized herbal treatments can offer significant relief.

These conditions are often multifaceted and require a comprehensive treatment strategy that addresses various aspects of the condition. Herbs are selected not only for their specific actions related to the condition but also for their ability to support other body systems that may be impacted by the condition or its conventional treatments.

The Importance of Personalization

Personalization is at the heart of specialized herbal treatments. Each person's experience of a health condition is unique, influenced by factors such as their overall health, lifestyle, and genetic predispositions. A specialized herbal treatment that works for one person may not be as effective for another, even if they have the same condition.

This individualized approach requires a thorough assessment of the person's health, including their medical history, current health status, and lifestyle. It also requires an openness to adjusting the treatment plan based on the person's response to the herbs.

The Role of Diet and Lifestyle

In specialized herbal treatments, the role of diet and lifestyle is emphasized as an integral part of the healing process. Herbs are powerful, but their effects can be enhanced or hindered by the person's diet and lifestyle choices.

For instance, in treating a condition like irritable bowel syndrome, dietary changes to eliminate trigger foods are often necessary alongside herbal treatments to reduce inflammation and support digestive health. Similarly, in conditions like anxiety or insomnia, lifestyle changes such as stress management techniques and establishing a regular sleep routine are essential components of the treatment plan.

Safety and Efficacy in Specialized Treatments

While specialized herbal treatments offer powerful healing possibilities, they also come with a responsibility to ensure safety and efficacy. This involves not only choosing the right herbs but also using them at the right dosages and ensuring they are of high quality.

Herbalists must also be aware of potential contraindications and interactions, particularly when herbs are used alongside conventional medications. Monitoring the person's response to the treatment and making adjustments as necessary is crucial to ensuring the safety and effectiveness of the treatment.

Specialized herbal treatments represent a profound aspect of herbal medicine. They offer the promise of targeted, effective healing for specific health conditions, grounded in a deep understanding of herbal pharmacology, the holistic nature of health, and the unique needs of each individual.

HERBAL RECIPES FOR SPECIFIC CONDITIONS

In the expansive world of herbal medicine, the creation of targeted remedies for specific health conditions is an art form that combines deep knowledge, experience, and intuition. This subchapter teaches herbal recipes specifically formulated to address particular health conditions. These recipes represent a synthesis of traditional knowledge and modern understanding, showcasing the power of herbs to provide relief and foster healing when tailored to specific needs.

Creating Targeted Herbal Remedies

The process of creating herbal recipes for specific conditions is a meticulous one. It involves selecting herbs not only for their primary therapeutic properties but also for their ability to work synergistically to enhance healing. Each recipe is crafted with an understanding of the underlying causes of the condition it aims to treat, and the herbs are chosen to address these root issues.

Herbal Remedies for Digestive Disorders

Digestive disorders, ranging from acid reflux to irritable bowel syndrome, can be effectively managed with specific herbal remedies.

1. **Acid Reflux Relief Tea**: A soothing blend of marshmallow root, slippery Elm bark, and chamomile can be used to create a tea that provides relief from acid reflux. The mucilaginous properties of marshmallow and slippery elm coat and protect the digestive tract, while chamomile reduces inflammation and eases discomfort.

2. **Irritable Bowel Syndrome (IBS) Tonic**: A combination of peppermint, fennel, and ginger can be used to create a tonic for IBS. Peppermint relaxes the smooth muscles of the digestive tract, fennel reduces bloating and gas, and ginger enhances digestive function.

Formulations for Respiratory Conditions

Herbs offer effective remedies for various respiratory conditions, including asthma and bronchitis.

3. **Asthma Relief Syrup**: A syrup made from elecampane, licorice root, and turmeric can benefit individuals with asthma. Elecampane acts as an expectorant, licorice has soothing properties, and turmeric's anti-inflammatory action can help reduce asthma symptoms.

4. **Bronchitis Herbal Tea**: A tea blending mullein, coltsfoot, and thyme can provide relief in cases of bronchitis. Mullein and coltsfoot help in expelling mucus, while thyme serves as a powerful antimicrobial agent.

Herbs for Skin Conditions

Specific herbs can be particularly beneficial in treating skin conditions such as eczema and acne.

5. **Eczema Healing Salve**: A salve made from calendula, chickweed, and plantain can be effective for eczema. These herbs have soothing, anti-inflammatory properties and promote skin healing.

6. **Acne Spot Treatment**: A topical treatment using Tea tree oil, Witch hazel, and green tea can be effective against acne. Tea tree oil has antimicrobial properties, Witch hazel acts as an astringent, and green tea reduces inflammation.

Mental Health and Herbal Support

Herbs play a significant role in managing mental health issues like anxiety and depression.

7. **Anxiety-Reducing Elixir**: A blend of lemon balm, passionflower, and lavender can create a calming elixir for anxiety. These herbs work synergistically to reduce stress and promote relaxation.

8. **Depression Relief Tincture**: St. John's Wort, combined with rosemary and lemon balm, can form a tincture beneficial for mild to moderate depression. St. John's Wort is well-known for its antidepressant properties, while rosemary and lemon balm support mood and cognitive function.

Herbal Remedies for Women's Health

Herbs can be specifically formulated to address various women's health issues, from menstrual cramps to menopausal symptoms.

9. **Menstrual Cramp Relief Tea**: A tea made from Cramp bark, ginger, and raspberry leaf can offer relief from menstrual cramps. Cramp bark eases uterine spasms, ginger alleviates pain, and raspberry leaf tones the uterine muscles.

10. **Menopause Symptom Soother**: A blend of black cohosh, sage, and red clover can help soothe menopausal symptoms. Black cohosh is effective for hot flashes, sage reduces sweating, and red clover helps balance hormones.

These herbal recipes represent the fusion of Barbara O'Neill's teachings with the rich tradition of herbalism. Each recipe is a testament to the potential of herbs to address specific health conditions in a targeted and effective manner. These formulations, while grounded in traditional knowledge, are also adaptable and can be tailored to meet the unique needs of each individual.

TECHNIQUES FOR COMBINING HERBS

The technique of combining herbs is akin to a culinary chef masterfully blending flavors to create a harmonious dish. Just as in cooking, the practice of combining herbs in therapeutic formulations is a delicate balance of understanding individual properties, interactions, and the desired therapeutic outcome. This subchapter explores the techniques of combining herbs, deep into the principles of herbal synergy, balance, and the creation of effective, holistic remedies.

The Foundation of Herbal Synergy

At the core of combining herbs is the principle of synergy, where the combined effect of the herbs is greater than the sum of their individual parts. O'Neill encourages thoughtfulness to formulation where each herb is selected not only for its own merits but also for how it complements and enhances the actions of other herbs in the blend.

1. **Understanding Herb Categories**: In crafting herbal combinations, it's crucial to understand different categories of herbs such as carminatives (like ginger and fennel), demulcents (such as slippery elm and marshmallow root), adaptogens (like ashwagandha and ginseng), and nervines (such as lemon balm and lavender). Understanding these categories aids in selecting herbs that work harmoniously to target various aspects of a condition.

2. **Complementary Actions**: When combining herbs, it's important to consider how their actions complement each other. For example, in a formula for digestive aid, combining a soothing demulcent like marshmallow root with a carminative like peppermint can address multiple facets of digestive discomfort.

Balancing Herbal Formulas

Balance is key in herbal combinations. This involves considering the energetics of the herbs (warm, cool, dry, moist) and ensuring that the formula is balanced in a way that matches the individual's constitution and the nature of their ailment.

1. **Energetic Balancing**: For instance, if using warming herbs like ginger in a formula, it may be balanced with cooler herbs

like peppermint to prevent overheating and irritation, especially in individuals with a warmer constitution.

2. **Dosage Ratios**: Balancing also involves adjusting the ratios of each herb in the formula. More potent herbs may be used in smaller quantities, while milder herbs may form the bulk of the formula.

Layering Herbal Effects

Layering involves combining herbs in a way that their effects unfold sequentially or target different aspects of a condition. This technique is particularly useful in complex conditions where multiple body systems are affected.

1. **Sequential Unfolding**: In a sleep aid formula, for instance, an initial layer of fast-acting nervines like lavender can be combined with deeper-acting, longer-lasting herbs like valerian to ensure both immediate relaxation and sustained sleep support.

2. **Multi-System Targeting**: For comprehensive immune support, a combination of an immediate immune stimulant like echinacea can be layered with a deeper, long-term immune modulator like astragalus.

Harmonizing Herbs and Reducing Adverse Effects

Combining herbs can also serve to harmonize the formula, reducing the potential for adverse effects, and enhancing tolerability.

1. **Mitigating Irritation**: Herbs with potent actions might be combined with soothing herbs to mitigate any potential irritation. For instance, a strong laxative herb like senna can be

combined with a soothing demulcent like marshmallow to prevent intestinal irritation.

2. **Enhancing Digestibility**: Bitter herbs that stimulate digestion, like gentian, can be combined with carminative herbs like cardamom or fennel to enhance digestibility and prevent potential discomfort like gas or bloating.

Creating Target-Specific Formulas

In creating target-specific formulas, understanding the primary and secondary actions of herbs is essential. This involves choosing a primary herb or herbs that directly address the main symptom or condition and supporting herbs that assist or amplify the primary herb's actions.

1. **Primary and Supportive Herbs**: In a formula for respiratory health, mullein may be the primary herb for its expectorant properties, supported by thyme for its antimicrobial action and licorice for its soothing effect on irritated mucous membranes.

2. **Layered Support**: In addressing a condition like anxiety, a primary herb such as ashwagandha, an adaptogen, can be supported by secondary herbs like passionflower and hops that provide immediate calming effects.

The art of combining herbs is a complex yet immensely rewarding aspect of herbal medicine. It involves a deep understanding of individual herbs, their energetics, actions, and interactions. The techniques of creating synergy, achieving balance, layering effects, harmonizing formulas, and crafting target-specific combinations are essential tools in the herbalist's repertoire.

TAILORING TREATMENTS FOR INDIVIDUAL NEEDS,

The focus on tailoring treatments to meet individual needs is paramount. This cancels the one-size-fits-all mentality often found in conventional medicine, recognizing the uniqueness of each individual's body, lifestyle, and health condition. This subchapter examines the art and science of customizing herbal treatments, a process that requires a deep understanding of the individual as a whole, their environment, and how different herbs can be used synergistically to address specific health concerns.

Understanding the Individual as a Whole

The cornerstone of O'Neill's approach is the understanding that each person is an intricate combination of physical, emotional, mental, and environmental factors. This understanding is crucial in customizing herbal treatments.

1. **Comprehensive Health Assessment**: The process begins with a comprehensive health assessment, which includes not only the individual's physical symptoms but also their emotional state, dietary habits, lifestyle, and environmental factors. For instance, in treating insomnia, the approach considers potential stressors, dietary habits, and lifestyle choices alongside physical symptoms.

2. **Personal Health History and Genetic Predispositions**: A detailed personal health history, including any familial health patterns or genetic predispositions, is also taken into account. This information can provide insights into the individual's inherent health strengths and vulnerabilities.

Incorporating Lifestyle and Dietary Considerations

O'Neill stresses that effective herbal treatment goes beyond just prescribing herbs. It involves incorporating lifestyle and dietary changes that support the healing process.

1. **Dietary Modifications**: Nutritional guidance is tailored to support the therapeutic action of herbs and address specific health issues. For example, an anti-inflammatory diet may be recommended alongside herbs for conditions like arthritis.

2. **Lifestyle Adjustments**: Recommendations on lifestyle adjustments such as exercise, sleep, stress management, and exposure to natural environments are integral to the treatment plan. These adjustments are tailored to complement the action of the herbs and enhance overall well-being.

Tailoring Herbal Formulations

Creating a herbal formulation to meet an individual's needs is a nuanced process that involves selecting herbs based on their specific actions and how they interact with each other and the individual's condition.

1. **Selecting Primary and Supportive Herbs**: The formulation typically includes a primary herb that directly addresses the main health concern and supportive herbs that assist in the healing process. For example, in a formula for hypertension, hawthorn may be the primary herb for its cardiovascular benefits, supported by calming herbs like lavender to address stress, a contributing factor to high blood pressure.

2. **Consideration of Herb Energetics**: The energetics of herbs; whether they are warming or cooling, drying or moistening, are considered to ensure the formula aligns with

the individual's constitution and current state. A person with a hot, fiery constitution, for instance, may require cooling and calming herbs.

Monitoring and Adjusting Treatments

Tailoring treatments is an ongoing process that involves careful monitoring and adjustments as needed.

1. **Regular Follow-ups and Adjustments**: Regular follow-up consultations are essential to assess the effectiveness of the treatment and make any necessary adjustments. The herbal formulation may be modified based on the individual's response and changes in their condition.

2. **Responsive and Dynamic Treatment Plans**: The treatment plan is dynamic and responsive, evolving as the individual's health needs change. This approach ensures that the treatment remains effective and relevant.

Tailoring treatments for individual needs is a meticulous and compassionate process. It involves a deep understanding of the individual as a whole, thoughtful creation of herbal formulations, and ongoing monitoring and adjustments.

Interactive Elements for Readers to Consider Personalization of Treatments

The personalization of herbal treatments is not just the prerogative of practitioners; it involves active participation from those seeking healing. This subchapter lights up the interactive elements that individuals can consider to personalize their own herbal treatments. This process empowers individuals to engage more deeply with their healing journey, integrating their unique needs, experiences, and responses into their treatment plans.

Self-Assessment as a Tool for Personalization

The first step in personalizing herbal treatment is self-assessment. This involves individuals taking stock of their health status, lifestyle, and specific health concerns.

1. Health and Symptom Journaling: Keeping a health and symptom journal can be an invaluable tool. This record helps track daily health experiences, symptom patterns, dietary habits, and emotional states. For instance, noting digestive discomfort in relation to meals can help pinpoint triggers and guide the selection of digestive-supportive herbs.

2. **Body Constitution Analysis**: Understanding one's body constitution (such as in Ayurvedic doshas or Traditional Chinese Medicine elements) can guide the choice of herbs. Individuals can evaluate their constitution through questionnaires or consultations with practitioners, selecting herbs that balance their specific constitution.

Engaging with Herbal Selection

In personalizing treatment, individuals can engage actively in the selection of herbs, guided by their understanding of their health needs and the properties of different herbs.

1. Research and Education: Educating oneself about different herbs and their properties is key. Resources like books, reputable online platforms, and workshops can provide valuable information on herbal actions, indications, and contraindications.

2. **Sensory Engagement with Herbs**: Direct engagement with herbs through sensory experiences smelling, tasting, and even growing them, can help individuals understand and connect with the herbs they choose to use. This connection can guide intuitive choices in herbal selection.

Incorporating Lifestyle and Environmental Factors

Personalization also involves considering one's lifestyle and environment, as these can significantly impact the effectiveness of herbal treatments.

1. **Lifestyle Considerations**: Factors such as stress levels, sleep patterns, and physical activity should be considered when choosing herbs. For example, individuals with high stress might benefit from adaptogenic herbs, while those with sleep issues might find nervine herbs more beneficial.

2. **Environmental Influences**: The environment, including climate, pollution levels, and seasonal changes, can influence health and the effectiveness of herbs. Individuals can choose herbs that counteract environmental stressors they are exposed to.

Seeking Professional Guidance When Needed

While personalization encourages self-involvement, recognizing when to seek professional guidance is important.

1. **Complex Health Conditions**: In cases of complex health conditions or when using potent herbs, consulting with a professional herbalist or healthcare provider is advised to ensure safety and effectiveness.

2. **Interpreting Responses**: Professionals can help interpret responses to herbs, especially in distinguishing between healing

reactions and adverse effects, and make necessary adjustments in treatment plans.

The personalization of herbal treatments is a deeply interactive process that places individuals at the center of their healing journey. It encompasses a blend of self-assessment, engaged learning, consideration of lifestyle and environmental factors, interactive decision-making, and responsive   personalization not only enhances the efficacy of herbal treatments but also fosters a deeper connection with the healing power of herbs and a greater understanding of one's own body and health.

CHAPTER 5: HOLISTIC HERBAL REGIMENS

This chapter unfolds comprehensively the holistic herbal medicine, where herbs are not merely agents of symptomatic relief but catalysts of comprehensive wellness. It goes deeper into how herbs can be integrated into daily life to support and enhance overall health, harmonize the body's systems, and nurture a deep connection between the individual and the natural world.

The Philosophy of Holistic Herbalism

At the heart of holistic herbal regimens lies the philosophy that human health is an intricate balance of physical, emotional, mental, and spiritual well-being. This philosophy, deeply ingrained in O'Neill's teachings, views the body as a coherent whole, where each part is intimately connected and where balance and harmony are essential for true health.

1. Holistic Approach to Health: Holistic herbalism approaches health not as a series of isolated symptoms but as a dynamic state of balance. It acknowledges that factors such as lifestyle, diet, emotional state, and environmental conditions all play a crucial role in health and well-being.

2. Herbs as Holistic Agents: In this view, herbs are seen not only as substances with medicinal properties but as holistic agents that interact with the body's systems in a multifaceted way. They offer benefits that extend beyond the physical, touching on emotional and spiritual dimensions of health.

Integrating Herbs into Daily Life

A key aspect of holistic herbal regimens is the integration of herbs into daily life. This practice goes beyond the occasional use of herbal remedies to address specific ailments and incorporates herbs as a regular part of maintaining health and preventing disease.

1. Daily Herbal Infusions: Incorporating herbal infusions or teas into daily routines is a simple yet effective way to reap the benefits of herbs. Herbs like chamomile, peppermint, or tulsi can be consumed regularly to support digestion, manage stress, and boost immunity.

2. **Herbal Foods and Supplements**: Integrating herbs into food, whether through culinary herbs like rosemary and thyme or through supplements like turmeric capsules, is another aspect of holistic regimens. This approach allows for a consistent and enjoyable way to include herbs in one's diet.

Supporting Various Body Systems

Holistic herbal regimens focus on supporting various body systems in a balanced manner. This involves using herbs that target specific systems while maintaining overall balance.

1. Digestive System Support: Herbs like ginger, fennel, and dandelion can be used to support digestive health, aiding in digestion, and ALLEVIATING common digestive issues.

2. **Nervous System Support**: Adaptogenic herbs such as ashwagandha and Holy basil play a key role in supporting the nervous system, helping the body manage stress and maintain emotional balance.

3. **Immune System Enhancement**: Echinacea, elderberry, and astragalus are examples of herbs that can be used to strengthen the immune system, particularly during times of increased risk of illness.

Harmonizing Body and Mind

Holistic herbal regimens also emphasize the harmonization of body and mind. This involves using herbs that not only address physical symptoms but also contribute to mental and emotional well-being.

1. Herbs for Mental Clarity and Focus: Ginkgo biloba and Gotu kola are herbs known for their ability to enhance mental clarity and focus, making them valuable in a holistic regimen that addresses cognitive health.

2. **Herbs for Emotional Well-being**: St. John's Wort, lavender, and lemon balm are herbs that can be particularly beneficial in managing mood and promoting emotional well-being.

Seasonal Herbal Practices

The holistic approach recognizes the importance of aligning herbal practices with the rhythms of nature, including the changing seasons.

1. Seasonal Detoxification: Herbs like milk thistle and burdock can be used for detoxification during seasonal transitions, such as spring or fall, to help cleanse the body and prepare it for the coming season.

2. **Adapting to Seasonal Needs**: The choice of herbs can also be adapted to meet the body's changing needs with the seasons, such as using warming herbs like ginger in the winter and cooling herbs like peppermint in the summer.

Chapter 5 unfolds the rich landscape of holistic herbal regimens, where herbs are seamlessly woven into the fabric of daily life, supporting health in a comprehensive and harmonious way. This offers a pathway to enduring health and wellness, emphasizing balance, integration, and the alignment with the natural rhythms of the body and the environment. It represents a paradigm shift from viewing herbs as mere remedies to embracing them as integral companions in the journey towards holistic health and well-being.

CREATING HOLISTIC TREATMENT PLANS

Embarking on the creation of holistic treatment plans is an exploration into a deeply integrative approach to health and wellness. This method transcends the mere alleviation of symptoms, focusing instead on cultivating optimal health by addressing the physical, emotional, mental, and spiritual aspects of an individual. This subchapter shows the art and science of developing integral treatment plans, emphasizing the importance of a personalized, comprehensive approach that harmonizes the body with its natural processes and the surrounding environment.

Incorporating Complementary Therapies

Holistic treatment plans may also integrate complementary therapies that align with O'Neill's holistic philosophy.

1. **Physical Therapies**: Practices such as massage, acupuncture, or chiropractic care may be included to address physical aspects of health, like pain relief or structural alignment.

2. **Mind-Body Practices**: Mind-body interventions like mindfulness, biofeedback, or guided imagery are often incorporated to support mental and emotional health.

Creating holistic treatment plans is a deeply thoughtful and individualized process. It encompasses a comprehensive understanding of the individual's health matrix, integrating tailored dietary and lifestyle changes, personalized herbal regimens, and complementary therapies. Regular monitoring and adaptation are key to ensuring the plan's effectiveness. Such a holistic treatment plan does more than address specific health issues; it nurtures overall well-being, aligns the individual with their natural state of health, and empowers them on their journey to holistic wellness.

UNDERSTANDING HOW DIFFERENT REMEDIES WORK TOGETHER

The synergy of remedies is not just a beneficial occurrence but a central concept. This subchapter explores the intricate interplay between different herbal remedies and how they work together to create a total healing effect. It is an in-depth examination of the principles of synergy, where the combined action of herbs is greater than their individual effects, and how this synergy can be harnessed to create more effective and comprehensive treatment plans.

Balancing Herbal Actions

The concept of balancing different actions of herbs is crucial in creating effective synergistic blends.

1. **Complementary Actions**: Herbs with complementary actions are often combined to enhance the overall effect. For instance, a calming herb may be paired with a mood-lifting herb in a formula designed for emotional balance.

2. **Counterbalancing Side Effects**: If one herb in a blend has potential side effects, another herb with counterbalancing properties can be included to mitigate these effects. For example, if a diuretic herb may potentially deplete potassium, it may be combined with a potassium-rich herb.

Layering Herbs for Sustained Effects

Layering herbs in a treatment plan involves using different herbs at different times or stages of treatment for a more sustained therapeutic effect.

1. **Immediate vs. Long-Term Relief**: Some herbs provide immediate relief of symptoms, while others work more gradually to address the underlying causes. A layered approach might involve using both types for immediate relief and long-term healing.

2. **Sequential Herb Use**: In some cases, different herbs may be used in succession. For example, an acute inflammatory condition may first be treated with anti-inflammatory herbs, followed by tonifying herbs to rebuild strength.

Creating Harmonious Blends

The creation of harmonious herbal blends requires an understanding of the energetic qualities and flavors of herbs, as well as their medicinal properties.

1. **Energetic Qualities**: Herbs have energetic qualities such as warming, cooling, drying, or moistening. A harmonious blend considers these qualities to create a balanced formula that aligns with the individual's constitution and the nature of their condition.

2. **Flavor Profiles and Medicinal Properties**: The flavors of herbs (bitter, sweet, pungent, etc.) often correlate with specific medicinal properties. Understanding these correlations can guide the creation of blends that are both effective and palatable.

The Role of Herbal Adjuvants

In herbal blending, adjuvants are substances that enhance the effectiveness of the primary herbs in the blend.

1. **Enhancing Bioavailability**: Some adjuvants can increase the bioavailability of key compounds in the primary herbs, making them more effective.

2. **Facilitating Delivery**: Adjuvants can also help in the delivery of the herbal constituents to specific tissues or systems in the body.

Understanding how different remedies work together is an exploration of the delicate art of synergy, balance, layering, harmony, and personalization. It is a deeper dive into the intelligent and thoughtful combination of herbs to create remedies that are not just effective in alleviating symptoms but are transformative in promoting overall health and well-being.

BALANCING HERBAL TREATMENTS WITH LIFESTYLE CHANGES

This subchapter advocates balance between herbal treatments and lifestyle changes. It illustrates how such a fusion not only amplifies the healing properties of herbs but also fosters an environment within the body that is conducive to long-lasting health and wellness.

Dietary Modifications to Enhance Herbal Efficacy

Diet plays a critical role in the efficacy of herbal treatments. The right nutritional choices can enhance the therapeutic effects of herbs, while poor dietary habits can diminish them.

1. **Nutrient-Rich Diet for Herbal Support**: A diet rich in vitamins, minerals, and antioxidants supports the body's natural healing processes and can enhance the efficacy of herbal treatments. Foods high in these nutrients can help in tissue repair, immune function, and overall vitality, providing a foundation for herbs to work more effectively.

2. **Avoiding Dietary Inhibitors**: Certain foods can inhibit the absorption or effectiveness of herbal remedies. For instance, highly processed foods, excessive caffeine, and sugar can interfere with the body's ability to absorb and utilize the beneficial compounds in herbs.

Incorporating Physical Activity into Herbal Regimens

Physical activity is a complementary aspect of herbal regimens. Regular exercise can enhance the effectiveness of herbal treatments by improving circulation, boosting mood, and enhancing overall energy levels.

1. **Types of Exercise**: The type of exercise recommended is based on the individual's health condition and treatment goals. For instance, gentle exercises like yoga or tai chi may be more suitable for those with chronic pain or stress-related conditions.

2. **Exercise as a Potentiator of Herbal Efficacy**: Regular physical activity can potentiate the effects of herbs by improving metabolic functions, enhancing detoxification processes, and boosting immune function.

Stress Management Techniques

Stress management is crucial in holistic herbal therapy, as stress can often exacerbate health conditions or hinder the healing process.

1. **Mind-Body Techniques**: Techniques such as meditation, deep breathing, and mindfulness can be effectively combined with herbal treatments to manage stress. These practices can help mitigate the impact of stress on the body and enhance the overall effectiveness of herbal remedies.

2. **Herbs and Stress Reduction**: Certain herbs known for their adaptogenic or calming properties can be more effective when combined with stress-reduction techniques, offering a comprehensive approach to managing stress-related conditions.

Integrating Adequate Rest and Sleep

Adequate rest and quality sleep are essential components that complement herbal treatments. Good sleep enhances the body's natural healing processes and allows herbal remedies to work more effectively.

1. **Herbs for Sleep Support**: Herbs that promote relaxation and sleep, such as valerian or chamomile, can be complemented by good sleep hygiene practices to maximize their effectiveness.

2. **Routine and Sleep Environment**: Establishing a regular sleep routine and creating a conducive sleep environment are lifestyle changes that can significantly impact the effectiveness of sleep-supportive herbs.

Environmental and Social Considerations

The individual's environment and social interactions also play a role in herbal therapy. A supportive environment and positive social connections can enhance the healing process.

1. **Creating a Healing Environment**: This may involve making changes to one's living space to reduce toxins, increase comfort, and promote relaxation, thereby creating an environment that supports wellness.

2. **Social and Emotional Support**: Engaging in supportive social relationships and community activities can positively impact mental and emotional health, complementing the effects of herbal treatments.

Balancing herbal treatments with lifestyle changes acknowledges the interconnectedness of physical, emotional, and environmental factors. This method extends the efficacy of herbs beyond their immediate effects, incorporating dietary and lifestyle modifications, physical activity, stress management, adequate rest, and a supportive environment into the treatment plan. This, not only addresses the symptoms but also fosters an overall state of health and well-being, embodying the true essence of holistic healing.

REITERATING KEY PRINCIPLES FROM O'NEILL'S HOLISTIC APPROACH

Holistic health, a concept passionate to Barbara O'Neill, is a philosophy that integrates the physical, emotional, mental, and spiritual aspects of an individual, aiming not just to alleviate illness but to promote overall vitality and wellness. This subchapter revisits the key principles of O'Neill, elucidating how these tenets form the bedrock of a truly integrative and transformative healing journey.

The Interconnectedness of Body, Mind, and Spirit

One of the foundational principles of O'Neill is the recognition of the interconnectedness of the body, mind, and spirit in health and healing.

1. **Holistic View of Health**: Health is perceived not just as the absence of disease but as a state of complete physical, mental, and social well-being. This view recognizes that imbalances in one aspect of health can affect the entire system.

2. **Mind-Body Connection**: O'Neill emphasizes the impact of mental and emotional states on physical health. Stress, anxiety, and negative emotions can manifest as physical symptoms, while positive emotions and mental resilience can enhance physical health.

Prevention as a Primary Goal

Prevention is as important as treatment. This principle is about proactively maintaining health and preventing illness before it manifests.

1. **Lifestyle as Preventive Medicine**: Adopting a healthy lifestyle is a cornerstone of preventive health. This includes nutritious eating, regular physical activity, adequate rest, and stress management.

2. **Herbs for Prevention**: Certain herbs are used not just for treatment but also for their preventive benefits. For instance, adaptogens are used to enhance the body's resistance to stress, and antioxidants are used to prevent cellular damage.

The Importance of Nutrition

Nutrition plays a central role in O'Neill's holistic approach. The adage "you are what you eat" underpins the belief that food can be medicine.

1. **Whole Foods Over Supplements**: Emphasis is placed on obtaining nutrients from whole foods rather than supplements. A diet rich in vegetables, fruits, whole grains, lean proteins, and healthy fats provides essential nutrients for health and well-being.

2. **Dietary Adaptation to Individual Needs**: Diets are tailored to individual needs, preferences, and health conditions. For example, anti-inflammatory diets may be recommended for conditions like arthritis, while blood-sugar-balancing diets may be advised for diabetes.

The Role of Herbal Medicine in Healing

Herbal medicine is more than a means to treat illness; it's a way to support and enhance overall health.

1. **Herbs as Natural Healers**: Herbs are valued for their natural healing properties and their ability to work in harmony with the body's own healing capabilities.

2. **Personalized Herbal Therapy**: Herbal treatments are personalized, taking into account the individual's unique health condition, lifestyle, and preferences. This customization ensures that herbal therapy is aligned with the person's specific needs.

Embracing Natural Rhythms and Cycles

O'Neill advises to live in harmony with nature's rhythms and cycles, believing that aligning with these natural patterns promotes health and well-being.

1. **Seasonal Living**: This includes adapting diets, activities, and even herbal remedies according to the seasons. For instance, lighter, cooling foods and herbs may be favored in summer, while warming, nourishing foods and herbs may be preferred in winter.

2. **Circadian Rhythms**: Respecting the body's natural circadian rhythms, especially in terms of sleep-wake cycles, is crucial for maintaining health. Disruptions to these rhythms can lead to various health issues.

Stress Management and Emotional Well-being

Managing stress and nurturing emotional well-being are key aspects of O'Neill's philosophy.

1. **Techniques for Stress Reduction**: Practices such as meditation, yoga, and deep breathing are recommended not just as relaxation techniques but as integral parts of maintaining holistic health.

2. **Herbs for Mental Health**: Herbs that support mental and emotional health, such as St. John's Wort for mild depression and Lemon Balm for anxiety, are used within the context of a broader strategy that includes lifestyle changes and emotional therapies.

Detoxification and Cleansing

Detoxification is another principle based on the belief that cleansing the body of toxins is essential for optimal health.

1. **Natural Detoxification Methods**: These include dietary changes, increased water intake, herbal detox formulas, and practices like sauna or steam baths to promote toxin elimination.

2. **Gentle, Sustainable Approaches**: O'Neill gives needs for gentle, sustainable detoxification methods that support the body's natural detoxification processes, rather than aggressive or extreme detox regimes.

Revisiting the key principles of Barbara O'Neill brings into focus the depth and breadth of holistic health. It underscores the importance of viewing health as an integrated state of physical, mental, and spiritual well-being, and of aligning with nature's rhythms and cycles.

Chapter 6: Herbal Detoxification and Cleansing

The concept of detoxification and cleansing, particularly through the use of herbal remedies, is a fundamental aspect. This chapter prioritizes the world of herbal detoxification and cleansing, and explores the intricate ways in which herbs can be used to purify and rejuvenate the body, emphasizing the importance of these processes in maintaining health and vitality.

The Philosophy of Detoxification in Herbal Medicine

Detoxification in herbal medicine is based on the principle that the body's natural healing processes can be enhanced by eliminating toxins and impurities that accumulate due to various factors such as diet, environmental pollutants, and stress.

1. **Holistic View of Detoxification**: Unlike the often aggressive detoxification methods popularized in mainstream culture, herbal detoxification is viewed holistically. It is seen not just as a physical cleansing process but as an opportunity to rejuvenate the body, mind, and spirit.

2. **Supporting Natural Body Processes**: The focus is on supporting the body's natural detoxification processes; primarily the liver, kidneys, digestive system, skin, and lungs, rather than forcibly expelling toxins.

Understanding Toxins and Their Impact on Health

A comprehensive understanding of what constitutes toxins and how they impact health is crucial in the context of herbal detoxification.

1. **Types of Toxins**: Toxins can come from external sources like pollutants, chemicals, and heavy metals, or internal sources like metabolic by-products. Understanding these sources is key to effectively addressing them through detoxification.

2. **Impact on Health**: Accumulation of toxins can lead to various health issues, including fatigue, digestive problems, skin conditions, and more serious chronic illnesses. The goal of detoxification is to alleviate these conditions by removing the source of the problem.

Herbs in Detoxification and Cleansing

Certain herbs have properties that make them particularly effective in aiding detoxification and cleansing.

1. **Liver-Supporting Herbs**: Herbs such as milk thistle, dandelion, and turmeric are known for their liver-supporting properties. They help enhance liver function, which is crucial in the detoxification process.

2. **Kidney Cleansing Herbs**: Herbs like uva ursi, cranberry, and nettle support kidney health and assist in the elimination of waste and excess water from the body.

Diet and Nutrition in Herbal Detoxification

Diet plays a significant role in supporting the body's detoxification processes, working in tandem with herbal remedies.

1. **Detoxification Diet**: A diet rich in fruits, vegetables, whole grains, and lean proteins provides the necessary nutrients and antioxidants to support the body during detoxification. Certain

foods like leafy greens, beets, and garlic are particularly beneficial in a detox diet.

2. **Hydration**: Adequate hydration is essential during detoxification. Water helps flush out toxins and supports kidney function. Herbal teas can also be a beneficial part of a hydration strategy during detox.

The Role of Digestive Health in Detoxification

A healthy digestive system is key to effective detoxification. Many herbs used in detoxification directly support digestive health.

1. **Digestive Aids**: Herbs such as ginger, peppermint, and fennel aid digestion and help alleviate issues like bloating and gas, which can be common during detoxification.

2. **Fiber**: Dietary fiber is essential in a detox diet as it helps bind to toxins and facilitate their elimination through the digestive tract. Herbs with high fiber content, like psyllium husk, can be incorporated into the diet for this purpose.

Customizing Herbal Detoxification Regimens

Herbal detoxification regimens should be tailored to individual needs, taking into account factors such as health status, lifestyle, and personal preferences.

1. **Personalized Herbal Selection**: The selection of herbs for detoxification should be based on the individual's specific health needs and goals. For instance, someone with skin issues might focus on herbs that support skin health in addition to general detoxification herbs.

2. **Duration and Intensity**: The duration and intensity of a detoxification regimen can vary. Short-term, intensive detox programs may be suitable for some, while others may benefit more from a longer, gentler detoxification process.

This chapter presents a comprehensive view of herbal detoxification and cleansing, integral to health. It emphasizes the importance of viewing detoxification as a supportive process that enhances the body's natural healing capabilities, rather than an aggressive expulsion of toxins. Through a combination of carefully selected herbs, supportive dietary and lifestyle practices, and personalized treatment plans, herbal detoxification and cleansing can be a powerful tool in achieving and maintaining optimal health.

METHODS FOR HERBAL DETOX AND CLEANSING ROUTINES

The practice of detoxification and cleansing is not just a trend, but a profound method of purifying and rejuvenating the body. This subchapter underscores the specific methods for implementing herbal detox and cleansing routine. It explores the various ways in which herbs can be utilized in detoxification processes, emphasizing their roles in supporting the body's natural detoxifying organs and systems, and enhancing overall health and vitality.

Foundation of Herbal Detoxification

Herbal detoxification is grounded in the understanding of herbs as natural facilitators of the body's detoxification processes. It involves employing herbs in a way that supports and enhances the body's innate ability to cleanse itself.

1. **Supporting Natural Detox Organs**: The primary focus is on supporting organs like the liver, kidneys, and digestive system, which are pivotal in the body's natural detoxification process. Herbs such as milk thistle for the liver and dandelion for the kidneys are often used.

2. **Gentle Cleansing**: The emphasis is on gentle cleansing rather than harsh detox methods. This involves using herbs that naturally stimulate the body's detoxification pathways without causing stress or depletion to the system.

Herbal Detox Tea Routines

One of the most common methods of herbal detoxification is through the use of detox teas. These teas are formulated with a blend of herbs known for their cleansing properties.

1. **Daily Detox Teas**: A daily detox tea might include herbs like green tea, nettles, and burdock root. This tea can be consumed once or twice daily as a gentle way to support the body's ongoing detoxification.

2. **Targeted Detox Teas**: For more targeted detox needs, such as liver cleansing, a tea blend might include herbs like milk thistle, dandelion root, and artichoke leaf. These teas can be consumed in short cycles, such as a week-long liver cleanse.

Herbal Detox Baths

Detox baths are another method of utilizing herbs for detoxification. They are beneficial for not just physical cleansing, but also for relaxation and stress reduction.

1. **Preparing Herbal Detox Baths**: A detox bath can be prepared by adding herbs like lavender, chamomile, or eucalyptus to bath water, either directly or in a muslin bag.

Epsom Saltss and essential oils may also be added for additional detoxifying and relaxing effects.

2. **Routine and Duration**: Detox baths can be taken once or twice a week as part of a regular detox routine. They are particularly beneficial when taken before bedtime to promote restful sleep.

Herbal Detox Supplements and Capsules

In some cases, herbal detoxification might involve the use of supplements or capsules, especially when specific, concentrated herbal actions are needed.

1. **Supplement Formulations**: Herbal supplements for detox may include concentrated extracts of herbs like turmeric, cilantro, or chlorella, known for their detoxifying properties. These are typically used in cases where a more intense detoxification is needed.

2. **Guidance and Duration**: The use of herbal supplements for detox should be guided by a knowledgeable practitioner, especially regarding dosage and duration, to ensure safety and effectiveness.

Herbal Juices and Smoothies

Incorporating detoxifying herbs into juices and smoothies is a refreshing and nourishing way to cleanse the body.

1. **Herbal Juice Recipes**: Juices can be made using detoxifying herbs and greens like parsley, cilantro, and wheatgrass, combined with fruits and vegetables such as apples, cucumbers, and celery.

2. **Smoothies with Herbal Additions**: Smoothies can include ingredients like spirulina, chlorella, or powdered greens, which offer detoxifying benefits in a more filling form.

THE ROLE OF DETOXIFICATION IN HOLISTIC HEALING

Detoxification is not just a process but a fundamental principle. This subchapter aligns the intricate role of detoxification within the holistic healing paradigm, emphasizing its significance. Here, detoxification is viewed not merely as a physical cleansing method, but as an integral part of a comprehensive approach to achieving and maintaining optimal health.

Detoxification as a Cornerstone of Holistic Health

Detoxification is seen as a cornerstone that supports the body's innate ability to heal and maintain balance.

1. **Natural Healing Facilitation**: Detoxification is perceived as a facilitator of the body's natural healing processes. By eliminating toxins and waste, it helps clear the path for the body's inherent self-repair mechanisms to function optimally.

2. **Restorative Process**: Beyond removal of toxins, detoxification is also about restoration and rejuvenation. It is seen as a vital process that helps reset the body's systems, enhancing overall vitality and energy.

The Role of Herbal Remedies in Detoxification

Herbal remedies are a central aspect of detoxification.

1. **Herbs for Organ Support**: Specific herbs are identified for their ability to support detoxification organs. For example, milk thistle for liver support or nettle for kidney health.

2. **Herbal Cleanses**: Short-term herbal cleanses, using teas or tinctures made from detoxifying herbs, are often recommended as a way to give the body's detoxification systems a boost.

Detoxification as a Preventative Measure

Detoxification is not only for those who are unwell; it is also seen as a preventive measure to maintain health and prevent disease.

1. **Routine Detox Practices**: Incorporating routine detox practices into one's lifestyle, such as regular detox weekends or seasonal cleanses, can help maintain optimal health and prevent the accumulation of toxins.

Holistic Detoxification and Chronic Disease

In cases of chronic disease, detoxification is tailored to support the body's healing processes, taking into consideration the specific needs and limitations of the individual.

1. **Gentle Detoxification**: For individuals with chronic conditions, a gentle approach to detoxification is often advocated, focusing on supporting rather than overburdening the body.

2. **Customized Detox Plans**: Detox plans for chronic disease patients are highly customized, taking into account the individual's condition, treatment regime, and overall health status.

The role of detoxification is comprehensive and multifaceted. It extends beyond the physical realm, encompassing emotional, mental, and environmental aspects of health. Detoxification is interwoven with nutrition, lifestyle, herbal medicine, and preventive health care, forming an integral part of a sustainable approach to health.

CHAPTER 7: LONG-TERM MANAGEMENT OF CHRONIC CONDITIONS

The management of chronic conditions represents one of the most challenging yet profoundly important aspects of healthcare. Long-term management of chronic conditions is above conventional methodologies, emphasizing an integrative and comprehensive strategy. This chapter is dedicated to exploring what is required for effectively managing chronic conditions over the long term.

The Holistic Perspective on Chronic Conditions

Chronic conditions, ranging from diabetes and heart disease to autoimmune disorders and chronic pain, pose unique challenges due to their persistent and often progressive nature.

1. **Understanding Chronic Conditions**: Chronic conditions are typically characterized by their long duration and generally slow progression. They often require ongoing management and can significantly impact an individual's quality of life.

2. **Holistic Approach**: The holistic approach to managing chronic conditions involves addressing the root causes and the interconnectedness of the body systems, rather than merely treating symptoms. This approach is grounded in the understanding that lifestyle, diet, emotional well-being, and environmental factors all play a critical role in the management of chronic diseases.

Dietary Interventions in Chronic Disease Management

Nutrition plays a crucial role in the management of chronic conditions, with dietary interventions tailored to address specific health concerns.

1. **Tailored Nutritional Plans**: Diet plans for chronic conditions are highly individualized. For instance, a low-glycemic diet may be prescribed for diabetes management, while an anti-inflammatory diet may be beneficial for autoimmune disorders.

2. **Functional Foods and Nutrients**: Emphasis is placed on incorporating functional foods that provide specific health benefits. These include foods rich in antioxidants, phytonutrients, omega-3 fatty acids, and fiber.

The Role of Herbal Medicine in Chronic Disease Management

Herbal medicine offers a complementary approach to managing chronic conditions, with herbs selected for their specific therapeutic properties.

1. **Supportive Herbal Therapies**: Herbs are chosen based on their ability to support the functioning of specific organs or systems affected by the chronic condition. For example, hawthorn for heart conditions or turmeric for its anti-inflammatory properties in autoimmune diseases.

2. **Safety and Efficacy**: The safety and efficacy of herbal remedies are paramount, especially considering the long-term nature of their use in chronic conditions. The potential interactions of herbs with conventional medications are carefully considered.

Customization and Flexibility in Management Approaches

The management of chronic conditions requires a high degree of customization and flexibility.

1. **Personalized Management Plans**: Each individual's management plan is made to meet their specific condition, lifestyle, preferences, and response to treatments. This customization ensures that the management approach is as effective and sustainable as possible.

2. **Ongoing Monitoring and Adaptation**: Chronic conditions often require ongoing monitoring and adaptation of management plans. Regular assessments help in fine-tuning the approach based on changes in the condition, lifestyle, and overall health.

Chapter 7 encapsulates a comprehensive and integrative approach to the long-term management of chronic conditions. It highlights the importance of a holistic perspective, which encompasses dietary interventions, lifestyle modifications, herbal medicine, mind-body practices, environmental considerations, and an overarching theme of customization and flexibility. This louds the importance of a harmonious balance between conventional medical treatments and holistic practices, offering a path to sustainable health and well-being for those living with chronic diseases.

MANAGING CHRONIC DISEASES WITH HERBAL REMEDIES

Managing chronic diseases with herbal remedies offers a pathway to wellness that is both natural and nurturing. This subchapter explores the selection, preparation, and application of various herbs, taking advantage of their potential to not only alleviate symptoms but also to address underlying imbalances that contribute to chronic conditions.

Herbalism in the Context of Chronic Disease Management

Herbal remedies are viewed not as mere substitutes for conventional medicines but as integral components of a comprehensive wellness strategy.

1. **Whole-Body Approach**: The use of herbs in managing chronic diseases is based on a whole-body approach. This method recognizes that chronic diseases often result from imbalances in the body and that herbs can help restore this balance.

2. **Herbs as Modulators**: Many herbs are known for their modulating effects on the body's systems. They can help regulate immune response, hormonal balance, and metabolic processes, which are often disrupted in chronic diseases.

Principles of Selecting Herbs for Chronic Conditions

The selection of herbs is a thoughtful process, grounded in an understanding of the specific needs of each chronic condition.

1. **Targeting the Root Causes**: Herbs are chosen not only for their ability to alleviate symptoms but also for their potential to target the root causes of the chronic condition. For example, adaptogenic herbs like Ashwagandha may be used in conditions like chronic fatigue syndrome for their ability to modulate stress responses.

2. **Considering Individual Differences**: Herbal selection also takes into account individual differences, including a person's age, constitution, and specific symptoms. This personalized approach ensures that the chosen herbs are more likely to be effective for the individual.

Preparing Herbal Remedies for Chronic Diseases

The preparation of herbal remedies is a crucial step in their effectiveness for managing chronic conditions.

1. **Formulations Tailored to Conditions**: Herbal remedies are often formulated as teas, tinctures, capsules, or extracts, depending on the condition being treated and the individual's preference. For instance, teas may be more appropriate for digestive disorders, while tinctures might be used for their concentrated effect in hormonal imbalances.

2. **Combinations for Synergistic Effect**: Herbs are often combined to create a synergistic effect, where the combined action of the herbs is greater than their individual effects. For example, a combination of anti-inflammatory herbs like Turmeric and immune-supporting herbs like Echinacea can be beneficial in autoimmune disorders.

Combining Herbal and Conventional Treatments

In many cases, herbal treatments for chronic diseases are used in conjunction with conventional medical treatments.

1. **Complementary Use**: Herbs can be used to complement conventional treatments, helping to alleviate side effects or enhance the overall effectiveness of medical therapies.

2. **Collaborative Care Approach**: It's important to adopt a collaborative care approach, where healthcare providers and herbal practitioners work together to provide the best possible care.

Safety and Contraindications

Safety is paramount when using herbal remedies, especially in the context of chronic diseases.

1. **Awareness of Contraindications**: It's vital to be aware of any contraindications or potential side effects of herbs, particularly in relation to any medications being taken.

2. **Professional Guidance**: Seeking guidance from a qualified herbalist or healthcare provider is recommended, especially when using herbs for serious chronic conditions.

Managing chronic diseases with herbal remedies is a complex but rewarding endeavor. It involves a thoughtful selection of herbs, careful preparation, integration with lifestyle changes, and a long-term commitment with regular monitoring. Through this, herbal remedies become powerful tools in the management of chronic conditions, offering hope and improved quality of life for many.

INCORPORATING LIFESTYLE AND DIETARY CONSIDERATIONS

This subchapter aims to unpack the nuances of integrating lifestyle and dietary modifications into the management of chronic conditions. We explore how these modifications are not just ancillary components but are central to a comprehensive strategy for long-term health management.

The Interplay of Diet and Chronic Disease Management

Dietary choices play a critical role in the management of chronic conditions. The foods we consume can either exacerbate or alleviate the symptoms and underlying causes of these conditions.

1. **Nutrition as Medicine**: O'Neill's views echo the concept of 'food as medicine', where dietary choices are seen as therapeutic tools. A nutrient-rich diet can provide the necessary support for the body to manage and possibly reverse certain chronic conditions.

2. **Anti-Inflammatory Diet**: Inflammation is a common thread in many chronic conditions. An anti-inflammatory diet, rich in fruits, vegetables, whole grains, healthy fats, and lean proteins, can help reduce inflammation and support overall health.

Customizing Diet to Individual Needs

Recognizing the uniqueness of each individual, dietary modifications should be personalized to fit one's specific health conditions, lifestyle, and even genetic predispositions.

1. **Individual Nutritional Requirements**: Tailoring diet plans to address individual deficiencies or excesses is crucial. This involves considering factors like age, gender, activity level, and specific health conditions.

2. **Cultural and Personal Preferences**: Dietary changes should also respect an individual's cultural background and personal preferences to ensure they are sustainable and enjoyable.

The Role of Herbal Nutrition

Incorporating herbs into the diet is a key aspect of O'Neill's approach to managing chronic conditions.

1. **Functional Herbs**: Certain herbs, due to their nutritional and medicinal properties, can be integrated into daily meals.

For instance, turmeric in cooking for its anti-inflammatory properties, or ginger for its digestive benefits.

2. **Herbal Supplements:** In some cases, herbal supplements may be used to provide concentrated nutrients that are difficult to obtain in sufficient quantities through diet alone.

Incorporating lifestyle and dietary considerations into the management of chronic conditions requires a comprehensive and personalized strategy. It involves not just focusing on symptom relief but addressing the underlying causes of the conditions, promoting overall well-being, and enhancing quality of life.

CHAPTER 8: WOMEN'S AND MEN'S HEALTH

Chapter 8 echoes the obscurity of women's and men's health, acknowledging the unique health concerns, challenges, and needs that arise due to differences in anatomy, hormonal fluctuations, and societal roles. This chapter offers an in-depth analysis of gender-specific health strategies, with emphasis on the importance of a personalized, empathetic, and inclusive approach to health care.

Understanding Gender-Specific Health Needs

Women's and men's bodies differ not only anatomically but also in how they react to disease, treatment, and lifestyle factors. Recognizing and addressing these differences is crucial for effective health management.

1. **Biological and Hormonal Variances**: Women and men experience different health risks and challenges due to biological differences, particularly hormonal variations. These differences can significantly impact physical health, mental well-being, and disease risk.

2. **Gender-Specific Diseases and Conditions**: Certain health conditions are unique or more prevalent in either women or men. For example, women face specific reproductive health issues such as menstrual disorders, polycystic ovary syndrome (PCOS), and menopause, while men are more prone to conditions like prostate enlargement and certain heart diseases.

Holistic Health in Women's Care

The holistic approach to women's health encompasses a broad spectrum of care, from reproductive health to general wellness, and acknowledges the impact of life stages such as menstruation, pregnancy, and menopause.

1. **Reproductive Health**: A holistic approach to reproductive health includes not only addressing physical symptoms but also considering emotional and mental health aspects. It involves managing conditions like menstrual irregularities, fertility issues, and menopausal symptoms with a combination of lifestyle modifications, nutritional support, and natural therapies.

2. **Preventive Care and Wellness**: Preventive care in women's health focuses on nutrition, exercise, stress management, and regular health screenings. Lifestyle interventions are tailored to reduce the risk of common women's health issues like breast cancer, osteoporosis, and autoimmune diseases.

Men's Health: Beyond the Physical

In men's health, a holistic approach extends beyond physical ailments to encompass mental and emotional well-being, often addressing the societal stigma around men's emotional health.

1. **Prostate Health and Cardiovascular Disease**: Key areas in men's health include prostate health, where conditions like benign prostatic hyperplasia (BPH) and prostate cancer are of concern, and cardiovascular health, as men are at a higher risk for heart diseases.

2. **Mental Health and Stress Management**: Acknowledging and addressing mental health issues, which are often underreported in men, is crucial. Stress management, emotional well-being, and addressing lifestyle factors like alcohol consumption and smoking are integral parts of a holistic men's health strategy.

Nutrition and Dietary Needs

The nutritional needs of women and men vary based on hormonal differences, metabolic rates, and risk of certain diseases. Tailoring diet to these needs is a key aspect of holistic health.

1. **Women's Nutritional Focus**: For women, dietary focus may include calcium and iron due to risks of osteoporosis and anemia, particularly during certain life stages like pregnancy and post-menopause.

2. **Men's Nutritional Focus**: Men's diets may need to emphasize heart-healthy foods rich in omega-3 fatty acids, fiber, and plant sterols to mitigate the risk of heart disease.

Exercise and Physical Activity

Physical activity is essential for both women and men, but the focus and type of exercise might differ based on specific health goals and physiological differences.

1. **Exercise for Women**: Exercise routines for women might focus more on strength training to combat the risk of osteoporosis, along with cardiovascular exercises for overall heart health.

2. **Exercise for Men**: Men's exercise regimens may emphasize cardiovascular health, weight management, and muscle building, considering the higher prevalence of obesity and heart disease.

Lifestyle Factors Influencing Health

Lifestyle factors play a significant role in both women's and men's health, impacting everything from hormonal balance to mental well-being.

1. **Stress and Its Management**: Understanding and managing stress is vital, as it can exacerbate gender-specific health issues such as hormonal imbalances in women and hypertension in men.

2. **Work-Life Balance**: Achieving a balance between work and personal life is essential for maintaining overall health and wellness. This balance helps mitigate stress, improve mental health, and enhance life satisfaction.

Emotional Well-being and Social Support

Emotional health and social support systems are integral to holistic health, with gender-specific nuances.

1. **Emotional Health in Women**: Women might benefit from support systems

that address the emotional aspects of menstrual health, childbirth, menopause, and balancing societal roles.

2. **Emotional Health in Men**: For men, creating safe spaces for expressing emotions and addressing mental health issues is key. This approach challenges the traditional norms that often discourage men from seeking help for emotional issues.

By integrating gender-specific nutritional needs, exercise regimens, lifestyle factors, and emotional health considerations, this approach provides a more effective and personalized pathway to health and wellness.

ADDRESSING HEALTH ISSUES THROUGH HERBAL REMEDIES

Addressing health issues with herbal remedies is a practice steeped in the understanding of the natural healing power of plants. This subchapter scans the intricate process of using herbal remedies to address a range of health issues. Here, we explore the selection, application, and integration of herbal remedies into health care, highlighting their role not just in symptom alleviation but in fostering overall health and well-being. This approach is grounded in a deep respect for the wisdom of nature and the body's innate capacity for healing.

Herbal Remedies: A Cornerstone of Holistic Health

Herbal remedies are viewed as more than mere supplements or alternatives to conventional medicine. They are considered vital tools that work in harmony with the body's natural processes.

1. **Nature's Pharmacy**: Herbs are rich in a variety of compounds that possess therapeutic properties. Each herb offers a unique profile of benefits, making them versatile tools in addressing a wide range of health issues.
2. **Whole-Person Approach**: The use of herbal remedies in this context is based on a holistic approach. This means considering the physical, emotional, and environmental factors that contribute to a health condition.

Addressing Women's Health Issues with Herbs

Herbal remedies can be particularly effective in addressing women's health issues, given their ability to balance hormones and address specific reproductive health concerns.

1. **Herbs for Menstrual Health**: Herbs like Chaste tree Berry (Vitex) and Red raspberry Leaf can be used to regulate menstrual cycles and alleviate symptoms like PMS.

2. **Menopause Support**: Herbs such as Black Cohosh and Sage have been traditionally used to manage menopausal symptoms, offering a natural alternative to hormone replacement therapy.

Herbal Remedies in Men's Health

In men's health, certain herbs have shown efficacy in addressing common issues such as prostate health and cardiovascular concerns.

1. **Prostate Health**: Herbs like Saw palmetto and Pygeum are known for their benefits in supporting prostate health and managing conditions like BPH.

2. **Heart Health**: Hawthorn Berry is an example of a herb used to support cardiovascular health, a common concern in men's health.

Managing Chronic Conditions with Herbs

Herbal remedies can play a significant role in the management of chronic conditions, offering a natural means to manage symptoms and improve quality of life.

1. **Herbs for Chronic Pain**: Herbs with analgesic properties, such as White Willow bark and Turmeric, can be used to manage chronic pain conditions.

2. **Supporting Digestive Health**: Herbs like Ginger and Peppermint can aid in digestive health, which is often a key component in managing chronic conditions.

Addressing health issues through herbal remedies is a practice that requires a deep understanding of herbal properties, individual health needs, and the integration of these remedies with lifestyle and dietary changes. By embracing the wisdom of herbal medicine and respecting the body's natural healing processes, this approach offers a compassionate, effective, and sustainable way to manage health issues and improve quality of life.

HERBAL SOLUTIONS FOR HORMONAL BALANCE AND REPRODUCTIVE HEALTH

Hormonal balance and reproductive health are pivotal aspects of overall well-being, deeply influencing physical, emotional, and mental health. Herbal solutions play a significant role in nurturing and maintaining this delicate balance. Here, we assess the integration of traditional wisdom and modern herbal practices, highlighting how specific herbs can be utilized to address a spectrum of hormonal and reproductive issues, with a focus on safety, efficacy, and the holistic harmony of the body.

Understanding Hormonal Balance

Hormonal balance is a dynamic and complex aspect of health, involving a delicate interplay of various hormones that regulate bodily functions.

1. **The Role of Hormones**: Hormones, acting as chemical messengers, play crucial roles in regulating metabolism, growth and development, tissue function, sexual function, reproduction, sleep, and mood.

2. Consequences of Imbalance: Hormonal imbalances can lead to a myriad of health issues, ranging from menstrual irregularities, infertility, weight gain, to mood swings and decreased energy levels.

Herbal Remedies for Women's Hormonal Health

In addressing women's hormonal health, specific herbs are known for their efficacy in balancing hormones and addressing reproductive health issues.

1. Chaste tree Berry (Vitex): Traditionally used for regulating menstrual cycles, Vitex is renowned for its ability to balance estrogen and progesterone levels, making it beneficial for conditions like premenstrual syndrome (PMS) and menopausal symptoms.

2. Red raspberry Leaf: Often used to strengthen the uterine lining and improve menstrual health, this herb is also popular among pregnant women for its uterine toning properties.

Herbs for Men's Hormonal Health

Men's hormonal health, particularly concerning testosterone levels and prostate health, can also be supported through specific herbs.

1. Saw palmetto: Widely used for prostate health, Saw palmetto can help in reducing the symptoms of benign prostatic hyperplasia (BPH) and may contribute to balancing testosterone levels.

2. Nettle Root: Nettle root supports prostate health and urinary functions. It is also thought to help in balancing male hormones and can be beneficial in reducing symptoms of BPH.

Supporting Fertility with Herbal Remedies

Fertility issues, affecting both men and women, can be addressed through a range of herbal remedies designed to enhance reproductive health.

1. **Maca Root**: Known for its hormone-balancing effects, Maca root is used to enhance fertility in both men and women. It is believed to improve sperm quality and quantity in men and regulate menstrual cycles in women.

2. **Shatavari**: Traditionally used in Ayurvedic medicine, Shatavari is considered a potent fertility-enhancing herb for women, believed to nourish the reproductive system and regulate menstrual cycles.

Managing Menopause and Andropause

Menopause in women and andropause in men are significant hormonal transition periods that can be managed effectively with herbal remedies.

1. **Black Cohosh**: Black Cohosh is commonly used for managing menopausal symptoms like hot flashes, mood swings, and sleep disturbances. It's thought to have estrogenic effects, helping to mitigate the decline in estrogen levels during menopause.

2. **Ginseng**: Ginseng is beneficial in managing andropause symptoms in men, including fatigue and decreased libido. It is also known for its overall energy-boosting properties.

Herbs for Thyroid Health

The thyroid gland plays a crucial role in hormonal health, and its dysfunction can lead to various health issues.

1. **Bladderwrack**: Rich in iodine, Bladderwrack is often used in herbal medicine to support thyroid function, particularly in cases of iodine deficiency.

2. **Ashwagandha**: This adaptogenic herb is known for its ability to support thyroid health, particularly in balancing thyroid hormones and improving symptoms of both hypothyroidism and hyperthyroidism.

The management of hormonal balance and reproductive health through herbal remedies, offers a natural, effective, and empathetic approach to healthcare. By imbibing the power of these natural remedies, individuals can navigate the complexities of hormonal and reproductive health with greater ease and efficacy.

REAL-LIFE EXAMPLES ILLUSTRATING THE APPLICATION IN GENDER-SPECIFIC HEALTH ISSUES

Exploring gender-specific health issues through the lens of real-life examples provides invaluable insights into the practical application of holistic health strategies. This subchapter avails a series of case studies and anecdotal experiences that illuminate the efficacy of tailored approaches in addressing health concerns unique to women and men. These narratives point out the role of personalized treatment, including herbal remedies, dietary adjustments, and lifestyle interventions. They offer a vivid illustration of how individualized care can lead to significant improvements in gender-specific health conditions.

Case Studies in Women's Health

1. **Polycystic Ovary Syndrome (PCOS)**: Sarah, a 28-year-old woman, struggled with irregular menstrual cycles, weight gain, and acne, classic symptoms of PCOS. Her treatment involved

a combination of dietary changes, including a low-glycemic diet and increased intake of whole foods, along with herbal remedies like Chaste tree Berry and Saw palmetto. This integrative approach not only regularized her menstrual cycles but also alleviated her acne and helped her manage her weight more effectively.

2. **Menopause Management**: Linda, a 52-year-old experiencing severe menopausal symptoms such as hot flashes, mood swings, and insomnia, found relief through a holistic regimen. Her plan included Black Cohosh and Evening Primrose Oil to manage hot flashes and mood swings, along with lifestyle modifications like regular yoga and mindfulness practices. These interventions significantly improved her quality of life during menopause.

Examples in Men's Health

1. **Benign Prostatic Hyperplasia (BPH)**: John, a 60-year-old man, faced urinary difficulties and discomfort due to BPH. His treatment included Saw palmetto and Nettle Root to alleviate urinary symptoms, complemented by dietary adjustments to include more vegetables and omega-3 fatty acids. Regular moderate exercise, particularly walking, also played a key role in his symptom management.

2. **Cardiovascular Health**: Mark, a 45-year-old with a family history of heart disease, integrated Hawthorn Berry into his routine as a preventive measure. Alongside, he adopted a heart-healthy diet rich in fiber, lean proteins, and healthy fats, and incorporated daily cardiovascular exercises into his lifestyle. His proactive approach led to improved cardiovascular health markers.

Integrating Herbal and Lifestyle Approaches

1. **Stress-Related Insomnia**: Emily, a 35-year-old woman, experienced insomnia linked to her high-stress job. Incorporating stress management techniques such as meditation and deep breathing, alongside herbal remedies like Valerian Root and Lemon Balm, she achieved significant improvements in her sleep quality and overall stress levels.

2. **Weight Management**: Alex, a 40-year-old man struggling with obesity, followed a holistic weight management plan. This included dietary changes focusing on reducing processed foods and sugars, increasing physical activity, and using herbs like Green Tea and Cayenne Pepper for their metabolic-boosting properties. His commitment to this comprehensive approach resulted in a sustainable weight loss.

Addressing Fertility Issues

1. **Female Fertility**: Rachel, a 30-year-old trying to conceive, faced irregular ovulation. Her holistic treatment plan involved dietary changes to balance hormones, regular acupuncture sessions, and herbs like Maca Root and Shatavari. These interventions helped normalize her ovulation and eventually led to a successful pregnancy.

2. **Male Fertility**: David, a 33-year-old with low sperm count, adopted a holistic approach to improve his fertility. This included dietary adjustments to increase antioxidants, regular exercise to boost testosterone levels, and herbs like Ashwagandha and Ginseng. Over time, his sperm count improved, aiding in his and his partner's journey to parenthood.

Holistic Approaches to Mental Health

1. **Depression in Women**: Anna, a 38-year-old woman, dealt with depression. Her holistic treatment included St. John's Wort for its mood-lifting properties, coupled with Omega-3 supplements and a diet rich in fruits and vegetables. Regular engagement in group fitness classes also provided her with both physical and social support.

2. **Anxiety in Men**: Kevin, a 42-year-old, experienced high levels of anxiety. His regimen included herbal remedies such as Passionflower and Kava, alongside mindfulness meditation and cognitive-behavioral therapy. These combined strategies helped him manage his anxiety more effectively.

These real-life examples demonstrate the profound impact of holistic health approaches in addressing gender-specific health issues. They illustrate that solutions tailored to individual needs, incorporating a blend of herbal remedies, dietary interventions, and lifestyle changes, can lead to significant health improvements. These narratives validate the principles of personalized care, maximizing the importance of understanding and addressing the unique health challenges faced by women and men.

CHAPTER 9: CHILDREN'S HERBAL REMEDIES

The utilization of herbal remedies in pediatric care presents a unique approach to addressing the health concerns of children. Unlike adults, children require more specialized and gentle care, considering their developing bodies and specific health needs. Chapter 9 investigates children's herbal remedies, drawing upon the principles of safety, efficacy, and age-appropriateness. The chapter aims to provide a comprehensive guide to using herbal treatments for common childhood ailments, balancing traditional wisdom with modern understanding.

The Distinctiveness of Children's Physiology

Children are not miniature adults; their bodies function differently and are in a continuous state of growth and development. This distinctiveness necessitates a careful approach when considering herbal remedies.

1. **Developing Immune System**: A child's immune system is still developing, making them more susceptible to infections but also offering a unique opportunity for building long-term immunity.

2. **Metabolic Rate and Dosage Considerations**: Children have a higher metabolic rate compared to adults, which affects how they process substances, including herbs. This necessitates careful consideration of dosages and formulations of herbal remedies.

Safe Use of Herbal Remedies in Children

Safety is paramount when using herbal remedies in pediatric care. The delicate nature of children's bodies requires a cautious approach to avoid any potential adverse effects.

1. **Choosing Safe Herbs**: Selecting herbs that are known for their safety and mildness in children is crucial. Herbs like Chamomile, known for its soothing properties, and Echinacea, used for immune support, are commonly used due to their safety profiles.

2. **Professional Guidance**: Consulting with a pediatrician or a qualified herbalist before administering herbal remedy for children is essential. They can provide guidance on appropriate herbs, dosages, and formulations suitable for children.

Common Childhood Ailments and Herbal Remedies

Various herbal remedies can be effectively used to treat common childhood ailments, from minor injuries and illnesses to chronic conditions.

1. **Colds and Flu**: Herbs like Elderberry and Echinacea are popular for their immune-boosting properties and can be used to shorten the duration of colds and flu.

2. **Digestive Issues**: For digestive discomforts such as colic or upset stomach, gentle herbs like Fennel and Peppermint can be beneficial.

Age-Appropriate Herbal Formulations

The formulation of herbal remedies for children must consider not only the appropriate dosages but also the palatability and administration method.

1. **Dosages for Children**: Herbal dosages for children are typically lower than for adults and need to be adjusted according to the child's age, weight, and health condition.

2. **Palatable Preparations**: Children are more likely to accept herbal remedies in pleasant-tasting forms, such as herbal syrups, glycerites, or teas sweetened with Honey (for children over one year of age).

Preventive Use of Herbal Remedies

In addition to treating specific ailments, herbal remedies can be used preventively in children to bolster their natural defenses and promote overall well-being.

1. **Immune Support**: Regular use of certain immune-supportive herbs, especially during cold and flu season, can help in building a child's resistance to infections.

2. **Gut Health**: Herbs that support digestive health can be used as a preventive measure, particularly for children with a tendency towards digestive issues.

This chapter emphasizes the importance of understanding the unique physiological and developmental needs of children when using herbal treatments. Through careful selection, safe formulation, and appropriate integration with diet and lifestyle, herbal remedies offer a natural and effective approach to addressing a wide range of childhood health issues. This serves as a guide for parents and caregivers in harnessing the gentle power of nature to nurture and maintain their child's health, underscoring the critical role of informed, cautious, and loving care in pediatric herbal therapy.

SAFE AND EFFECTIVE HERBAL TREATMENTS FOR CHILDREN

In the holistic approach to children's healthcare, the use of herbal treatments necessitates a careful balance between safety and efficacy. This subchapter tells of herbal remedies specifically tailored for children. This covers a range of herbal treatments suitable for various childhood ailments.

Principles of Herbal Treatment in Pediatrics

The application of herbal remedies in pediatrics involves several key guidelines to ensure they are both safe and effective.

1. **Gentleness is Key**: Herbs chosen for children are typically gentler and milder than those used for adults. The idea is to support rather than overpower the child's developing systems.

2. **Minimum Effective Dose**: The dosages used are carefully calculated based on the child's age, weight, and overall health condition, adhering to the principle of using the minimum effective dose to achieve the desired therapeutic effect.

Common Pediatric Ailments and Herbal Remedies

Various common childhood ailments can be safely and effectively treated with specific herbs, each chosen for their suitability in pediatric care.

1. **Respiratory Infections**: For common colds and mild respiratory infections, herbs like Elderberry, known for its immune-boosting properties, and Thyme, with its natural expectorant qualities, are often used. These herbs can be administered in the form of syrups or mild teas.

2. **Digestive Issues**: Digestive complaints such as colic, indigestion, and mild constipation in children can be managed with gentle herbs like Chamomile, known for its calming effect on the digestive system, and Fennel, which can relieve gas and bloating.

Preparations Suitable for Children

The form in which an herb is administered is as important as the herb itself, especially in pediatric care.

1. **Herbal Syrups and Glycerites**: These are often preferred for children due to their palatable taste. Herbal syrups can be made from a variety of herbs, depending on the condition being treated, and are sweetened in a natural and healthy manner.

2. **Infusions and Mild Teas**: Herbal teas, made from gentle herbs and sufficiently diluted, can be a comforting and effective way to administer herbal treatments to children.

Collaboration with Healthcare Professionals

Collaboration with pediatricians or professional herbalists is crucial when using herbal treatments, especially for more serious or chronic conditions.

1. **Integrative Approach**: Working with healthcare professionals ensures that the herbal treatments are part of an integrative approach, complementing any other medical treatments the child may be receiving.

2. **Professional Oversight**: Regular check-ups and consultations with healthcare professionals help in monitoring the child's progress and adjusting treatments as needed.

Sustainable and Ethical Sourcing of Herbs

The sustainability and ethical sourcing of herbs used in pediatric treatments are important considerations, aligning with the holistic principle of caring for the earth as well as the individual.

1. **Choosing Organic Herbs**: Whenever possible, choosing organic herbs free from pesticides and chemicals is recommended, as this ensures the purity and safety of the remedies given to children.

2. **Ethical Sourcing Practices**: Supporting ethical sourcing practices not only ensures the quality of the herbs but also contributes to the preservation of natural resources.

The use of safe and effective herbal treatments for children is a thoughtful process that requires careful consideration of the child's unique needs. It involves selecting appropriate herbs, preparing them in child-friendly forms, integrating them seamlessly into daily routines, and ensuring parental education and professional collaboration.

ADJUSTING DOSAGES AND FORMATS FOR PEDIATRIC USE

The adjustment of dosages and formats to suit the unique needs of children is a critical aspect of safe and effective treatment. The emphasis here is on understanding how children's physiology differs from adults and the implications this has for herbal medicine.

Fundamentals of Pediatric Herbal Dosage

Determining the correct dosage of herbal remedies for children is far more complex than simply reducing adult dosages. It requires an understanding of children's metabolic rate, body weight, age, and overall health.

1. **Age-Based Adjustments**: Dosage guidelines often vary significantly depending on the child's age. Infants and toddlers, for instance, require much lower doses compared to older

children, given their smaller body size and developing organ systems.

2. **Weight Considerations**: In many cases, dosages are calculated based on the child's weight. This approach ensures that the dosage is proportional to the child's physical size, a critical factor in the effective and safe use of herbal medicine.

Integrating Herbal Remedies into Children's Routines

Incorporating herbal remedies into a child's daily routine can enhance their acceptability and efficacy.

1. **Mealtime Integration**: Administering herbal remedies with meals or snacks can improve compliance in children. It can also aid in the digestion and absorption of the herbs.

2. **Creating Positive Associations**: Making the process of taking herbal remedies a positive experience can encourage adherence. This might involve creating a routine around remedy administration or pairing it with a favored activity.

Herbal Medicine as Part of a Holistic Health Approach

In pediatric care, herbal remedies are most effective when used as part of a holistic health approach, which includes diet, lifestyle, and emotional well-being.

1. **Balanced Diet**: A nutritious diet that supports a child's overall health can enhance the effectiveness of herbal remedies. This includes a diet rich in fruits, vegetables, whole grains, and adequate proteins.

2. **Healthy Lifestyle**: Adequate sleep, regular physical activity, and a stress-free environment contribute to the overall health of the child and the efficacy of the herbal treatments.

Professional Guidance and Collaboration

Working with healthcare professionals is vital, especially when using herbs to treat more serious or chronic conditions in children.

1. **Consulting with Pediatricians**: Regular consultations with a pediatrician ensure that the herbal treatments align with the child's overall healthcare plan.
2. **Collaboration with Herbalists**: Involving a professional herbalist can provide additional insights into the appropriate use of herbal remedies, ensuring they are tailored to the child's specific needs.

Adjusting dosages and formats of herbal remedies for pediatric use is a practice that demands meticulous attention to detail, a deep understanding of children's unique physiological needs, and a commitment to safety.

DISCUSSION ON COMMON MISCONCEPTIONS AND O'NEILL'S APPROACH TO PEDIATRIC HERBAL CARE

In pediatric herbal care, misconceptions abound, often stemming from a lack of understanding or misinformation about the nature and efficacy of herbal remedies for children. Addressing these misconceptions is crucial for fostering a safe and informed approach to pediatric herbalism. This subchapter aims to dispel these myths and elucidate the principles of safely incorporating herbal remedies into children's health care. By exploring O'Neill's approach, we gain a clearer understanding of how to effectively and responsibly use herbal treatments in pediatric care.

Common Misconceptions in Pediatric Herbalism

There are several widespread misconceptions regarding the use of herbal remedies in children, often leading to either undue skepticism or inappropriate use.

1. **"Herbs Are Completely Safe Because They Are Natural"**: One of the most prevalent myths is that all herbal remedies are inherently safe because they are natural. However, like all treatments, herbs can have side effects and interact with other medications. Recognizing that natural does not always equate to safe is crucial in pediatric herbal care.

2. **"Adult Herbal Remedies Can Be Directly Translated to Children"**: Another common misconception is that children can safely consume adult herbal remedies in smaller doses. This overlooks the specific physiological and developmental needs of children, potentially leading to ineffective or harmful dosing.

O'Neill's Approach to Dispelling Myths

Barbara O'Neill's approach to pediatric herbal care offers valuable insights into addressing these misconceptions.

1. **Emphasis on Safety and Appropriateness**: O'Neill stresses the importance of understanding the safety profile of each herb used in children, including potential side effects and interactions. Her approach involves thoroughly researching and understanding the herbs before recommending them for pediatric use.

2. **Customization of Herbal Remedies for Children**: O'Neill advocates for the customization of herbal remedies to suit the unique needs of children. This includes consideration of age-appropriate dosages, suitable formats for administration, and the child's specific health condition and overall constitution.

Responsible Use of Herbs in Children

Responsible use of herbal remedies in children involves several key practices.

1. **Start with the Least Invasive Options**: O'Neill's approach often involves starting with the least invasive herbal options, particularly those known for their gentle action and minimal side effects.

2. **Use of Culinary Herbs**: Incorporating common culinary herbs, which are generally milder and well-tolerated, can be an effective and safe way to introduce herbal treatments to children.

Overcoming Skepticism with Evidence-Based Practices

To overcome skepticism and build trust in pediatric herbal care, reliance on evidence-based practices is vital.

1. **Research and Clinical Evidence**: O'Neill encourages the use of herbs backed by research and clinical evidence, particularly those with a proven track record of safety and efficacy in children.

2. **Case Studies and Anecdotal Evidence**: Sharing successful case studies and anecdotal evidence, while not a substitute for scientific research, can provide practical insights into the effective use of herbs in pediatric care.

Herbal Education for Families

Educating families about the benefits and proper use of herbal remedies is a cornerstone of O'Neill's approach.

1. **Workshops and Resources**: Providing workshops, literature, and online resources can empower parents with the knowledge needed to safely use herbal remedies at home.

2. **Encouraging Informed Decision-Making**: Empowering parents to make informed decisions regarding their child's health care, including the use of herbal remedies, is a key aspect of O'Neill's educational approach.

Addressing common misconceptions in pediatric herbal care is crucial for the safe and effective use of herbal remedies in children. Barbara O'Neill's approach, characterized by an emphasis on safety, customization, and education, offers valuable guidance in this area. By dispelling myths, educating parents, and integrating herbal treatments with conventional care, a responsible and informed approach to pediatric herbalism can be achieved.

CHAPTER 10: MENTAL AND EMOTIONAL WELL-BEING

The pursuit of mental and emotional well-being is as vital as maintaining physical health, yet it often remains shrouded in less clarity and understanding. This chapter explores the world of mental and emotional health, recognizing it as an integral part of overall well-being. The focus here is on understanding, nurturing, and maintaining mental and emotional wellness through various natural and holistic methodologies. This exploration emphasizes the interconnectedness of the mind, body, and spirit, acknowledging that true health encompasses all aspects of human experience.

The Complexity of Mental and Emotional Health

Mental and emotional well-being is multifaceted, encompassing our thoughts, emotions, behaviors, and overall psychological state. It's a dynamic continuum, influenced by various internal and external factors.

1. **Understanding Emotional Health**: Emotional health refers to how well we manage our emotions and express them appropriately. It involves awareness, understanding, and acceptance of our feelings, and the ability to handle stress, adapt to change, and overcome challenges.

2. **Mental Health Spectrum**: Mental health includes our emotional, psychological, and social well-being. It influences how we think, feel, act, handle stress, relate to others, and make choices. Its state can range from flourishing to struggling to clinical mental illness.

Herbal Remedies in Mental Health

The use of herbal remedies in supporting mental and emotional well-being has been a practice for centuries. Rooted in traditional knowledge, these natural treatments offer an alternative or complement to conventional methods.

1. **Herbs for Stress and Anxiety**: Herbs such as Ashwagandha, Lavender, and Lemon Balm are renowned for their stress-relieving properties. They can be used to create a calming effect, reduce anxiety, and promote relaxation.

2. **Natural Mood Enhancers**: St. John's Wort, Rhodiola, and Saffron are some of the herbs known for their mood-enhancing properties. They have been traditionally used to alleviate symptoms of depression and improve emotional well-being.

Emotional Well-being in Different Life Stages

Mental and emotional health needs can vary significantly across different stages of life, requiring tailored approaches for children, adolescents, adults, and the elderly.

1. **Childhood and Adolescence**: During these formative years, the focus is on fostering healthy emotional development, resilience, and coping skills. Addressing issues like bullying, self-esteem, and academic stress is crucial.

2. **Adulthood and Aging**: In adults, managing work-life balance, family responsibilities, and societal pressures are key for mental health, while for the elderly, issues like loneliness, loss of independence, and cognitive decline take precedence.

The Role of Community and Social Connections

The impact of community and social connections on mental and emotional health cannot be overstated. A sense of belonging, community involvement, and strong social support networks are essential components of emotional well-being.

1. **Building Strong Social Ties**: Engaging in community activities, nurturing friendships, and maintaining close family ties can provide emotional support and a sense of belonging.

2. **Addressing Loneliness and Isolation**: In a world where loneliness and social isolation are increasing, creating opportunities for meaningful social interactions is more important than ever.

Overcoming Challenges to Mental Wellness

Confronting the challenges to mental and emotional health involves recognizing the barriers, be they societal stigma, lack of resources, or personal struggles, and finding ways to overcome them.

1. **Combating Stigma**: One of the biggest challenges in addressing mental health is the stigma associated with it. Education, open conversations, and advocacy are key to breaking down these barriers.

2. **Access to Resources**: Ensuring access to mental health resources, including counseling, therapy, and support groups, is essential for those struggling with mental and emotional issues.

Chapter 10 offers a comprehensive insight into the vast and complex domain of mental and emotional well-being. It underscores the necessity of a holistic approach that encompasses not just medical or therapeutic interventions but also considers lifestyle, nutrition, herbal remedies, social connections, and the overarching environment.

EXPLORING HERBS FOR MENTAL HEALTH AND STRESS RELIEF

The use of herbs for mental health and stress relief is pivotal. This subchapter looks into the depth of herbalism, focusing on herbs that have been traditionally and scientifically acknowledged for their benefits in enhancing mental well-being and alleviating stress. This exploration reveals how specific herbs can be incorporated into daily routines to support mental health, mitigate stress, and foster a balanced emotional state, all within the framework of holistic well-being.

Herbs for Alleviating Anxiety and Stress

Certain herbs are specifically valued for their calming and anxiolytic properties.

1. **Lavender (Lavandula angustifolia)**: Renowned for its soothing scent, Lavender is widely used for its ability to reduce anxiety and induce relaxation. Its essential oil, used in aromatherapy, or the dried herb in teas, can provide a calming effect on the nervous system.

2. **Chamomile (Matricaria recutita)**: Traditionally used as a mild relaxant, Chamomile is effective in soothing stress and easing anxiety. Its gentle nature makes it suitable even for children, often used to calm restlessness or anxiety.

Herbs for Depression and Mood Imbalances

Certain herbs have been recognized for their potential in managing depression and mood swings, offering natural alternatives or adjuncts to conventional treatment.

1. **St. John's Wort (Hypericum perforatum)**: Widely known for its antidepressant properties, St. John's Wort has been used for centuries to alleviate symptoms of mild to moderate depression. It is thought to work by increasing the levels of neurotransmitters in the brain.

2. **Rhodiola Rosea**: Rhodiola is an adaptogen, aiding the body in adapting to stress, and is known for its ability to enhance mood and alleviate depression. Its role in balancing the stress hormones makes it particularly useful for stress-induced mood swings.

Herbs for Cognitive Function and Mental Clarity

Enhancing cognitive function and mental clarity is another area where herbal remedies can be significantly beneficial.

1. **Ginkgo biloba**: Ginkgo is well-known for its ability to enhance cognitive function. It improves blood flow to the brain, which can help with memory retention, focus, and overall mental clarity.

2. **Gotu kola (Centella asiatica)**: Traditionally used in Ayurvedic and Chinese medicine, Gotu kola is reputed for its ability to improve mental function and is often used as a tonic for memory and concentration.

Adaptogenic Herbs for Stress Management

Adaptogenic herbs have a unique capacity to help the body resist and adapt to stress and exert a normalizing effect upon bodily processes.

1. **Ashwagandha (Withania somnifera)**: Ashwagandha is highly revered for its stress-relieving properties. It helps the

body cope with external stresses such as toxins in the environment and internal stresses such as anxiety and insomnia.

2. **Holy basil (Tulsi)**: Holy basil, known as Tulsi in Ayurvedic medicine, is another adaptogen that helps the body adapt to stress and maintain mental balance. It is also revered for its spiritual significance in many cultures.

Addressing Sleep Disorders with Herbs

Poor sleep quality is a common issue affecting mental health. Certain herbs can be effective in promoting restful sleep.

1. **Valerian Root (Valeriana officinalis)**: Valerian is often used for its sedative properties, effective in treating insomnia and improving sleep quality.

2. **Passionflower (Passiflora incarnata)**: Passionflower is another herb used for its sleep-inducing properties. It is particularly beneficial for those with insomnia related to anxiety.

The exploration of herbs for mental health and stress relief offers a comprehensive approach to managing mental well-being. By understanding and utilizing the therapeutic properties of specific herbs, and integrating them into a balanced lifestyle, one can effectively support mental and emotional health.

HOLISTIC METHODS FOR IMPROVING MENTAL AND EMOTIONAL WELLNESS

This subchapter reiterates various holistic strategies aimed at enhancing mental and emotional wellness. The focus here is not solely on treating symptoms but on nurturing the whole person; mind, body, and spirit. This approach recognizes the interconnectedness of various aspects of health and promotes a range of practices, from lifestyle changes and stress management techniques to natural therapies and community involvement.

Integrating Natural Therapies

The use of natural therapies, including herbal remedies, aromatherapy, and others, is a key aspect of improving mental and emotional wellness in a holistic way.

1. **Herbal Remedies**: Herbs like St. John's Wort, Ashwagandha, and Lavender can be used under professional guidance to address symptoms of stress, anxiety, and mild depression.

2. **Aromatherapy**: The use of essential oils, either through diffusers, baths, or topical application, can have a calming and uplifting effect on the mind and emotions.

Mind-Body Practices

Mind-body practices are central to O'Neill's holistic approach, emphasizing the interconnectedness of physical health with mental and emotional well-being.

1. **Yoga and Tai Chi**: These practices not only improve physical fitness but also enhance mental clarity, emotional balance, and stress resilience.

2. **Biofeedback and Mindfulness-Based Stress Reduction (MBSR)**: Techniques such as biofeedback and MBSR enable individuals to become more aware of their body's responses to stress and learn how to control them effectively.

Embracing Creativity and Recreation

Participation in creative and recreational activities is often overlooked but is vital in enhancing mental and emotional wellness.

1. **Creative Expressions**: Activities like painting, writing, or playing music provide an outlet for expressing emotions and can be incredibly therapeutic.

2. **Outdoor Activities and Nature Exposure**: Spending time in nature and engaging in outdoor activities can have a rejuvenating effect on both the mind and emotions.

Cultivating Positive Mindsets

O'Neill emphasizes the power of positive thinking and cultivating mindsets that support mental and emotional wellness.

1. **Practicing Gratitude**: Regularly practicing gratitude can shift focus from negative to positive aspects of life, enhancing overall emotional well-being.

2. **Cognitive Reframing**: Learning to reframe negative thoughts and perceptions into positive ones can significantly impact emotional health and resilience.

The methods for improving mental and emotional wellness offer a comprehensive and multi-faceted approach. This approach integrates physical health, stress management, social connections, natural therapies, mind-body practices, restful sleep, creative outlets, and positive mindsets into a cohesive strategy for mental and emotional health.

Reflective Questions or Exercises Applying Teachings to Personal Mental Health Scenarios

In the quest for mental and emotional well-being, self-reflection plays a pivotal role. This subchapter emphasizes the importance of reflective questions and exercises in applying teachings to personal mental health scenarios. These introspective practices are designed to deepen self-awareness, uncover underlying emotional patterns, and foster a proactive approach to mental health.

The Power of Self-Reflection in Mental Health

Self-reflection is a powerful tool in understanding and managing one's mental and emotional well-being. It involves looking inward, examining thoughts, feelings, and behaviors, and understanding their impact on one's life.

1. **Awareness of Emotional States**: Regular self-reflection helps in recognizing and acknowledging current emotional states, whether they are stress, anxiety, contentment, or joy. This awareness is the first step in managing emotions effectively.

2. **Understanding Thought Patterns**: Reflective practices aid in identifying recurrent thought patterns that may be contributing to mental health issues, such as tendencies toward negative or catastrophic thinking.

Reflective Questions for Personal Insight

Reflective questions are designed to provoke thought and insight into one's mental and emotional processes. They can be used as a part of daily journaling or during meditation.

1. **What are the predominant emotions I felt today, and what triggered them?**: This question helps individuals track their emotional responses and the triggers, enhancing emotional regulation.

2. **What thoughts tend to recur in my mind, and how do they affect my mood and behavior?**: This prompts introspection into habitual thought patterns and their impact on one's emotional state.

Exercises for Applying Holistic Teachings

Applying holistic teachings to one's life involves practical exercises that integrate these teachings into daily routines.

1. **Gratitude Journaling**: Keeping a gratitude journal, where one writes down things they are thankful for each day, can shift focus from negative to positive, enhancing overall well-being.

2. **Mindfulness Practice**: Engaging in mindfulness practices, such as mindful breathing or mindful walking, helps in staying present and reduces tendencies to ruminate on past or future worries.

Visualization and Affirmations

Visualization and affirmations are powerful tools in molding one's mental state and fostering a positive mindset.

1. **Positive Visualization**: Practicing visualization, where one imagines a positive outcome or a peaceful scenario, can have a calming effect and help in developing a positive outlook on life.

2. **Affirmations**: Repeating positive affirmations daily can help in rewiring the brain towards positive thinking and self-empowerment.

Reflective Exercises for Stress Management

Managing stress is crucial for mental health, and reflective exercises can be highly effective in this regard.

1. **Stress Diary**: Keeping a stress diary, where one notes down moments of high stress and their responses to these situations, can help in identifying patterns and triggers of stress.

2. **Relaxation Techniques**: Practicing relaxation techniques, such as progressive muscle relaxation or guided imagery, especially during times of high stress, can provide immediate relief and enhance long-term stress management skills.

Developing Emotional Resilience

Emotional resilience is the ability to adapt and bounce back from stress and adversity. Reflective exercises can help in building this resilience.

1. **Challenge and Change Perspective**: Encouraging oneself to view challenges as opportunities for growth and learning helps in developing resilience.

2. **Journaling for Resilience**: Writing about past challenges and how one overcame them can reinforce a sense of strength and resilience.

Self-Compassion Exercises

Self-compassion is fundamental to mental health, involving treating oneself with the same kindness and understanding as one would treat a friend.

1. **Self-Compassion Breaks**: Taking short breaks during the day to speak to oneself compassionately, especially during times of failure or difficulty, can enhance self-esteem and reduce self-criticism.

2. **Loving-Kindness Meditation**: Practicing loving-kindness meditation, where one directs feelings of love and kindness towards themselves and others, can foster an attitude of compassion and interconnectedness.

Addressing Mental Blocks and Barriers

Reflective questions and exercises can also help in identifying and addressing mental blocks and barriers that hinder emotional well-being.

1. **Identifying Limiting Beliefs**: Questions like "What beliefs are holding me back?" can help in recognizing and challenging limiting beliefs.

2. **Exploring Solutions**: Reflecting on questions like "What steps can I take to overcome these barriers?" encourages proactive problem-solving.

Reflective questions and exercises form an essential component of holistic mental health care. They offer a pathway for individuals to engage deeply with their emotional and mental processes, apply holistic teachings to their personal scenarios, and foster growth and healing. These practices encourage a journey of self-discovery, awareness, and transformation, leading to improved mental and emotional wellness.

CHAPTER 11: SEASONAL HERBAL REMEDIES

The concept of aligning healthcare practices with the rhythms of nature is deeply rooted and widely respected. This recognizes the dynamic interplay between our bodies and the changing seasons, advocating for the use of seasonal herbal remedies as a way to harmonize our internal health with the external environment. Chapter 11 offers a profound exploration into the world of seasonal herbal remedies, drawing from traditional wisdom and modern holistic practices. This involves the intricacies of selecting, preparing, and utilizing herbs that are particularly beneficial at different times of the year, thereby optimizing health and wellness in alignment with nature's cycles.

The Significance of Seasonal Changes in Health

Human health and wellness are intrinsically linked to the cycles of nature. Each season brings with it unique environmental changes that can impact physical and mental well-being.

1. **Impact of Seasons on Health**: The changing seasons can influence various aspects of health, including immune system function, mood, energy levels, and even susceptibility to certain health conditions. For instance, winter can bring about challenges in immune health and mood, while summer might stress hydration and heat-related issues.

2. **Seasonal Adaptation of the Body**: The human body naturally undergoes certain adaptations in response to seasonal changes. Understanding and supporting these adaptations through the use of appropriate herbal remedies can enhance health and well-being.

Spring: Detoxification and Renewal

Spring is often associated with renewal and detoxification, making it an ideal time to cleanse and rejuvenate the body after the winter months.

1. **Herbs for Detoxification**: Herbs like Dandelion, Nettle, and Milk Thistle are renowned for their detoxifying properties. They support liver function, aid in the elimination of toxins, and provide a refreshing start to the new season.

2. **Supporting Allergy Relief**: Spring is also the season of allergies for many. Herbs like Butterbur and Quercetin can be effective in easing allergy symptoms.

Summer: Energy, Hydration, and Vitality

During the warm summer months, the focus shifts to maintaining hydration, protecting the skin, and sustaining energy levels in the face of increased outdoor activity.

1. **Herbs for Hydration and Cooling**: Herbs such as Hibiscus, Mint, and Cucumber are perfect for their cooling and hydrating properties. They can be used in teas or infused waters to keep the body cool and hydrated.

2. **Natural Sun Protection and Skin Care**: Herbs like Green Tea and Aloe vera offer protective and soothing properties for the skin, which can be beneficial in addressing sun exposure and promoting skin health during summer.

Autumn: Immune Boosting and Preparation for Winter

Autumn is a transitional period, where strengthening the immune system becomes a priority in preparation for the colder months.

1. **Immune-Boosting Herbs**: Echinacea, Elderberry, and Astragalus are excellent for bolstering the immune system. Their use during autumn can help prepare the body for the upcoming winter.

2. **Herbs for Respiratory Health**: With the onset of colder weather, respiratory health becomes crucial. Herbs like Mullein, Thyme, and Licorice can support lung health and aid in respiratory function.

Winter: Immune Support and Mood Enhancement

Winter challenges include maintaining immune function and coping with reduced sunlight and its effects on mood and energy.

1. **Supporting Immune Health**: Continuing the use of immune-supportive herbs like Elderberry, Garlic, and Ginger can help maintain health during the winter months.

2. **Mood and Energy Support**: Herbs like St. John's Wort and Rhodiola
can be particularly useful in addressing seasonal affective disorder (SAD) and low energy levels often associated with the shorter days and longer nights of winter.

Seasonal Affective Disorder (SAD) and Herbal Remedies

The reduced sunlight in winter can lead to Seasonal Affective Disorder, a type of depression related to changes in seasons. Certain herbs can help alleviate its symptoms.

1. **St. John's Wort**: Known for its antidepressant properties, St. John's Wort can be beneficial for those experiencing mild to moderate SAD symptoms.

2. **Rhodiola Rosea**: An adaptogen, Rhodiola can help enhance mood and combat fatigue, making it suitable for combating the lethargy often associated with SAD.

Understanding Seasonal Diet and Herbal Integration

The integration of seasonal diets with herbal remedies is a key aspect of holistic health. Eating according to the season and complementing it with corresponding herbal remedies can optimize health.

1. **Seasonal Foods**: Consuming foods that are naturally available in each season can provide the body with nutrients that are particularly needed during that time.

2. **Harmonizing Diet with Herbs**: For example, incorporating light, detoxifying foods and herbs in spring aligns with the body's natural inclination towards cleansing after winter.

The Role of Environmental Factors

The change in environmental conditions with each season significantly impacts our health. Adjusting herbal remedies according to environmental changes is crucial for maintaining balance.

1. **Adapting to Humidity and Dryness**: In humid summers, astringent herbs like Witch hazel can be useful, while in dry winters, moisturizing herbs like Marshmallow root can be beneficial.

2. **Coping with Seasonal Allergens**: In seasons where allergens are prevalent, herbs that support the respiratory system and immune response can be particularly helpful.

Herbal Preparations According to Seasons

The method of preparing and consuming herbs can also vary with seasons to match the body's needs.

1. **Cold Infusions in Summer**: Cold infusions or herbal iced teas are ideal for summer, providing hydration and cooling effects.

2. **Warm Decoctions in Winter**: In winter, warm herbal decoctions and hot teas can provide warmth and boost immunity.

The use of seasonal herbal remedies, as part of a broader holistic approach to health, offers a profound way to align our bodies with the natural rhythms of the earth. By understanding and respecting the unique requirements of each season, and by utilizing herbs, diet, and lifestyle practices that resonate with these natural cycles, we can optimize our physical, mental, and emotional well-being throughout the year.

ADAPTING HERBAL TREATMENTS ACCORDING TO THE CHANGING SEASONS

The philosophy of adapting herbal treatments to the changing seasons is a fundamental aspect of holistic health care. This is a recognition that our health needs to evolve with the changing seasons, and therefore, the herbs we use for treatment and wellness should also vary correspondingly. Embracing the cyclical nature of the earth and its correlation with human health, this subchapter explores the adaptation of herbal treatments to different seasons and how this practice not only aligns with the body's natural rhythms but also enhances the efficacy of herbal remedies in promoting health and preventing illness.

The Rationale Behind Seasonal Herbal Adaptation

Understanding why and how the body's needs change with the seasons is key to effectively adapting herbal treatments.

1. **Seasonal Health Needs**: Each season brings with it unique environmental factors; temperature changes, humidity levels, allergens, and varying amounts of sunlight, all of which impact health differently. For instance, winter's cold can increase susceptibility to respiratory illnesses, while summer heat might stress hydration and skin health.

2. **Aligning with Natural Rhythms**: Adapting herbal treatments according to the seasons is about aligning with the body's natural rhythms. This approach helps in maintaining balance and harmony in the body, reducing the risk of seasonal health issues.

Understanding Herbal Energetics in Seasonal Context

Herbal energetics, the warming, cooling, drying, or moistening nature of herbs; play a crucial role in seasonal adaptation.

1. **Matching Energetics to Seasonal Needs**: Using herbs with energetics that match the seasonal needs of the body can enhance health and well-being. For example, cooling herbs are more suited for summer, while warming herbs are beneficial in winter.

2. **Individual Energetics**: It's also important to consider the individual's unique energetics and constitution when selecting herbs, as personal needs may vary even within a given season.

For instance, some individuals may require more moistening herbs in winter if they have a naturally dry constitution.

Seasonal Changes and Mental Health

The changing seasons also affect mental and emotional well-being, and adapting herbal treatments accordingly can be highly beneficial.

1. **Winter Blues and Herbal Mood Lifters**: In winter, shorter daylight hours can lead to Seasonal Affective Disorder (SAD). Herbs like St. John's Wort and Rhodiola can be helpful in uplifting mood.

2. **Stress and Relaxation**: During stressful seasons, such as the end-of-year holidays, herbs like Valerian and Chamomile can aid relaxation and stress relief.

Incorporating Seasonal Foods and Herbs

Integrating seasonal foods with herbal treatments enhances their effectiveness and supports overall health.

1. **Eating with the Seasons**: Consuming fruits and vegetables that are in season ensures a diet rich in necessary nutrients and aligns with the body's seasonal needs.

2. **Cooking with Herbs**: Incorporating culinary herbs and spices that are suited to the season, such as Basil in summer or Rosemary in winter, adds both flavor and health benefits to meals.

Preventive Health and Seasonal Herbalism

Using herbs seasonally is not only about treating existing health issues but also about preventive health care.

1. **Proactive Immune Support**: For example, starting immune-boosting herbs in the fall can prepare the body for the winter cold and flu season.

2. **Seasonal Cleansing**: Engaging in seasonal cleansing or detoxification rituals, using appropriate herbs, can help reset and rejuvenate the body.

Adapting Herbal Forms and Preparations with Seasons

The form in which herbs are used can also change with the seasons to better suit the body's needs.

1. **Teas and Infusions**: Light, cooling herbal teas are ideal for summer, while warm, spicy teas are comforting in winter.

2. **Topical Applications**: Depending on the season, different herbal salves, lotions, or oils can be used for skin care, such as cooling aloe-based lotions in summer or rich, moisturizing calendula cream in winter.

The adaptation of herbal treatments according to the changing seasons is a deep holistic approach to health care. It requires an understanding of the unique demands each season places on the body and the mind, and how various herbs can be used to meet these demands effectively. By aligning herbal remedies with the natural rhythms of the earth, not only can physical health be optimized, but mental and emotional well-being can also be significantly enhanced.

Season-Specific Wellness Tips and Remedies Reflecting O'Neill's Understanding of Nature's Rhythms

The changing seasons bring a diverse range of wellness challenges and opportunities. Acknowledging and aligning with nature's rhythms is crucial for maintaining optimal health throughout the year. This subchapter simplifies season-specific wellness tips and herbal remedies, drawing on O'Neill's profound understanding of how the cycles of nature impact our physical and mental well-being.

Adapting to Seasonal Changes in Lifestyle and Diet

Each season requires specific adjustments in lifestyle and diet to align with the body's changing needs.

1. **Sleep Adjustments**: Adapting sleep patterns to the changing length of days can help maintain the body's natural circadian rhythm. For instance, longer sleep hours might be beneficial in winter.

2. **Seasonal Eating**: Eating seasonally not only ensures a diet rich in necessary nutrients but also supports the body's natural dietary inclinations during different seasons.

Mindfulness and Emotional Health with Seasons

Being mindful of the emotional and mental shifts that accompany seasonal changes is crucial for holistic well-being.

1. **Acknowledging Seasonal Affective Disorder (SAD)**: Particularly in winter, it's important to recognize and address symptoms of SAD. Activities that foster light exposure, such as walks during daylight and light therapy, can be beneficial.

153

2. **Emotional Self-Care**: Engaging in activities that uplift spirits, such as connecting with loved ones, practicing self-care rituals, or pursuing hobbies, can help maintain emotional balance throughout the seasonal changes.

Herbal Support for Seasonal Affective Disorders

Certain herbs can be particularly effective in managing the emotional and psychological effects brought on by seasonal changes.

1. **Mood-Enhancing Herbs**: Herbs like St. John's Wort and Rhodiola can be used to manage mood swings and depressive symptoms, especially useful in seasons with reduced sunlight.

2. **Adaptogens for Stress**: Adaptogens like Ashwagandha and Holy basil can help the body adapt to seasonal stressors, maintaining mental and emotional equilibrium.

Seasonal Skin Care with Herbal Remedies

Adapting skin care routines to the changing seasons using herbal remedies can help maintain skin health and appearance.

1. **Hydration in Winter**: Using hydrating herbal remedies like Calendula or Aloe vera can prevent dry, chapped skin in winter.

2. **Cooling Remedies in Summer**: Herbal remedies with cooling properties, such as Cucumber or Witch hazel, can soothe and protect the skin during the hotter months.

Building Resilience to Seasonal Allergies

Seasonal allergies can be a significant issue during certain times of the year, particularly in spring and autumn.

1. **Herbs for Allergy Relief**: Incorporating herbs like Nettle, which has natural antihistamine properties, or Quercetin, can provide relief from allergy symptoms.

2. **Dietary Adjustments**: Consuming local Honey and incorporating anti-inflammatory foods can also help build resilience against seasonal allergies.

Cultural Practices and Seasonal Wellness

Many cultural practices around the world embrace the concept of aligning health practices with the seasons, offering valuable insights.

1. **Traditional Seasonal Practices**: Practices such as Ayurvedic seasonal routines or Traditional Chinese Medicine's alignment with seasonal energies can provide a deeper understanding of how to live in harmony with nature's rhythms.

2. **Community and Seasonal Festivities**: Participating in seasonal festivities and community activities can foster a sense of connection and well-being, aligned with the season's spirit.

Adapting herbal treatments and lifestyle practices according to the changing seasons is a profound way to maintain balance and harmony in both physical and mental health. This advocates for a responsive and dynamic way of caring for health. By tuning into the unique demands of each season and utilizing specific herbs, foods, and lifestyle practices, individuals can optimize their health and well-being throughout the year.

CHAPTER 12: INCORPORATING HERBS INTO DAILY LIFE

Incorporating herbs into daily life is a practice that dates back to ancient times, reflecting a deep connection between human health and the natural world. This chapter examines the art and science of integrating herbal remedies into everyday routines, a concept that is gaining renewed interest in modern holistic health practices. It addresses the practical aspects of selecting, preparing, and using herbs in a way that is both effective and harmonious with contemporary lifestyles.

The Relevance of Herbs in Modern Life

In the modern world, herbs offer not only health benefits but also serve as a means to slow down, reconnect with nature, and nurture a more mindful approach to health.

1. **Preventive Health**: Herbs offer a natural way to support the body's defenses, improve resilience to stress, and enhance overall vitality, aligning well with the preventive health paradigm.

2. **Accessibility and Sustainability**: With a growing emphasis on sustainable living, incorporating herbs into daily life also represents an environmentally friendly approach to health and wellness.

Herbs for Daily Wellness

Certain herbs are particularly well-suited for daily use, offering general wellness benefits without being overly potent or specific in action.

1. **Adaptogens for Stress**: Herbs like Ashwagandha, Holy basil, and Rhodiola are known for their adaptogenic properties, helping the body to manage stress more effectively.

2. **Digestive Aids**: Herbs such as Peppermint, Fennel, and Chamomile can be incorporated daily to support digestion and alleviate common digestive issues.

Incorporating Herbs into Family Health

Herbs can be safely and effectively incorporated into family health practices, offering natural options for everyday ailments.

1. **Children and Herbs**: Introducing mild and safe herbs to children, such as Chamomile for calming or Echinacea for immune support, can be a gentle way to address common health concerns.

2. **Educating Family Members**: Educating family members about the benefits and safe use of herbs encourages a holistic approach to health within the household.

Balancing Herbs with Lifestyle

For herbs to be most effective, they should be part of a balanced lifestyle that includes adequate sleep, exercise, and stress management practices.

1. **Holistic Health Approach**: Adopting a holistic approach to health where herbal remedies complement other health practices ensures a well-rounded and effective wellness strategy.

Incorporating herbs into daily life offers a holistic, natural, and enjoyable approach to health and wellness. By understanding the properties of different herbs and integrating them into daily routines, meals, family health practices, and even household products, individuals can greatly enhance their quality of life. Using herbs in daily life is not just about treating ailments; it's about nurturing a deeper connection with nature, fostering preventive health care, and enriching all aspects of personal and family well-being.

Everyday Uses of Herbs for Health and Wellness Following O'Neill's Lifestyle Recommendations

The use of herbs in daily life involves integrating these natural remedies into various aspects of our daily routines for health and wellness. This subchapter explores the practical, everyday applications of herbs. It emphasizes the philosophy that maintaining health is not just about reactive treatments but is deeply rooted in the proactive, daily integration of natural remedies and practices.

Herbal Supplements for Daily Health

For those seeking more concentrated benefits or specific therapeutic effects, herbal supplements can be incorporated into daily health routines.

1. **Daily Herbal Capsules or Tablets**: Supplements like turmeric capsules for inflammation, milk thistle for liver health, or ashwagandha for stress relief
can be taken as part of a daily supplement regimen.

2. **Quality and Source Considerations**: When choosing herbal supplements, it's important to consider the quality and

source, opting for products that are organic and sustainably sourced.

Herbal Teas for Hydration and Wellness

Herbal teas offer a delightful and healthful way to stay hydrated while enjoying the therapeutic benefits of various herbs.

1. **Custom Tea Blends**: Creating custom tea blends based on personal health needs and preferences can be a rewarding practice. For example, a blend of peppermint, ginger, and chamomile can aid digestion and soothe the stomach.

2. **Regular Tea Rituals**: Establishing a routine of herbal tea consumption, such as a calming chamomile tea before bed or a refreshing green tea in the morning, can be an enjoyable and healthful daily ritual.

Herbal Approaches to Immune Support

Strengthening the immune system is a key focus of holistic health, and daily use of certain herbs can be beneficial.

1. **Daily Immune Tonics**: Herbs like echinacea, astragalus, and elderberry can be used as tonics to boost the immune system, particularly during times when it is under stress, such as the cold and flu season.

2. **Incorporating Immune-Boosting Herbs in Meals**: Garlic, onions, and medicinal mushrooms can be included in daily meals for their immune-enhancing properties.

Herbs for Energy and Vitality

For those seeking natural ways to boost energy and vitality, certain herbs can be particularly effective.

1. **Adaptogenic Herbs for Energy**: Adaptogens like ginseng and rhodiola can help improve energy levels and resilience to stress.

2. **Herbal Smoothies and Juices**: Adding powdered or fresh herbs like spirulina, wheatgrass, or maca to smoothies or juices can provide a natural energy boost.

Herbs in Mindfulness and Meditation Practices

Integrating herbs into mindfulness and meditation practices can enhance their benefits.

1. **Burning Herbal Incense**: Herbs such as sage, cedar, and sweetgrass can be used as incense during meditation or mindfulness practices, aiding in grounding and focus.

2. **Herbal Essential Oils in Meditation**: Applying or diffusing essential oils during meditation can help deepen the practice and promote relaxation.

Incorporating herbs into daily life is a practice that enhances overall wellness, offering natural solutions for a range of health concerns. By weaving herbs into nutrition, stress management, immune support, and other aspects of daily living, individuals can tap into the vast healing potential of the plant world.

This represents a shift from reactive healthcare to a more balanced, holistic way of living, where health is nurtured daily through natural, simple, and effective means. By adopting this, individuals can foster a lifestyle that is in harmony with nature, sustainable, and deeply enriching.

CLEAR, ACTIONABLE PLAN FOR READERS TO START INCORPORATING HERBS DAILY

Incorporating herbs into daily life is a practice that can significantly enhance overall health and well-being. However, for many individuals, knowing where to start can be a challenge. This subchapter provides a clear and actionable plan to guide readers in integrating herbal remedies into their daily routines. The aim is to make the use of herbs accessible, practical, and effective, enabling readers to harness the full potential of these natural healers in a way that is sustainable and enjoyable. This comprehensive guide outlines step-by-step methods to seamlessly incorporate herbs into various aspects of daily life, from dietary habits to wellness routines, ensuring a holistic approach to health.

Step 1: Understanding Herbal Basics

Before integrating herbs into daily life, gaining a basic understanding of different herbs and their properties is essential.

1. **Research Common Herbs**: Start by researching common herbs and their health benefits. Familiarize yourself with herbs like ginger for digestion, lavender for relaxation, and echinacea for immune support.

2. **Learn About Herbal Safety**: Educate yourself on the safe usage of herbs, understanding potential side effects and interactions, especially if you are taking prescription medications.

Step 2: Setting Intentions and Goals

Define clear intentions and goals for incorporating herbs into your life. This will guide your choices and help you stay focused.

1. **Identify Health Goals**: Determine what health aspects you want to improve with herbs; whether it's boosting immunity, improving sleep, managing stress, or enhancing digestion.

2. **Set Realistic Expectations**: Understand that herbs are a complementary approach and may take time to show results. Set realistic expectations for your herbal journey.

Step 3: Starting with Simple Herbal Integrations

Begin by integrating herbs into your daily routines in simple, manageable ways.

1. **Herbal Teas**: Start your day with a cup of herbal tea suited to your health goals. For example, peppermint tea can be refreshing and aid digestion, while chamomile tea can be calming.

2. **Cooking with Herbs**: Incorporate culinary herbs like rosemary, thyme, and basil into your cooking. Use turmeric and ginger liberally for their anti-inflammatory properties.

Step 4: Incorporating Herbal Supplements

If specific health needs require more potent herbal interventions, consider herbal supplements.

1. **Choose Quality Supplements**: Opt for high-quality, organic herbal supplements from reputable sources.

2. **Start with Low Doses**: Begin with lower doses to see how your body responds and gradually increase as needed.

Step 5: Developing a Daily Herbal Routine

Establish a daily routine that incorporates herbal practices consistently.

1. **Morning Rituals**: Include herbal tonics or smoothies in your morning routine. Consider Aloe vera juice for digestive health or a green smoothie with spirulina for energy.

2. **Evening Wind-Down**: Create an evening routine with relaxing herbal teas or a warm bath infused with lavender or Epsom Saltss for relaxation.

Step 6: Personalizing Herbal Choices

Tailor your herbal selections to your unique health needs and preferences.

1. **Consider Personal Health Conditions**: Choose herbs that specifically address your individual health concerns. For instance, if you have chronic stress, adaptogenic herbs like ashwagandha may be beneficial.

2. **Preference and Taste**: Select herbs that you enjoy in terms of taste and aroma. This increases the likelihood of you sticking with your herbal routine.

Step 7: Creating Herbal Infusions and Decoctions

Learn to make basic herbal infusions and decoctions to extract the maximum benefits from herbs.

1. **Making Herbal Teas**: Steep herbs like chamomile or peppermint in hot water to make soothing teas.

2. **Preparing Decoctions**: For tougher herbs like roots and bark, simmer them in water for a longer period to make a decoction.

Step 8: Exploring Topical Applications

Explore the use of herbs topically for skin and hair care, as well as for muscle and joint health.

1. **Herbal Oils and Salves**: Create or purchase herbal oils and salves for topical application. For example, use arnica oil for bruises or aches, and calendula salve for skin irritations.

2. **Herbal Baths and Soaks**: Add herbs or essential oils like Epsom Saltss, lavender, or rosemary to baths for a relaxing and therapeutic experience.

Step 9: Integrating Herbs into Household Products

Replace some chemical-laden household products with herbal alternatives for a healthier living environment.

1. **Natural Cleaning Products**: Use herbs like thyme and lavender in homemade cleaning products for their natural antiseptic properties.

2. **Herbal Air Fresheners**: Create natural air fresheners using essential oils or dried herbs to enhance the ambiance of your home.

Step 10: Growing Your Own Herbs

If space allows, growing your own herbs can be a rewarding way to ensure a fresh, readily available supply.

1. **Starting a Herb Garden**: Begin with easy-to-grow herbs like basil, mint, and parsley. Even a small windowsill garden can provide a range of herbs.

2. **Harvesting and Storing**: Learn how to harvest and store herbs correctly to maintain their potency and freshness.

Step 11: Keeping a Herbal Journal

Documenting your herbal journey can be insightful and help track progress and responses.

1. **Record Experiences and Observations**: Note down how you feel after using certain herbs, any changes in health conditions, and recipes or preparations you've tried.

2. **Adjusting and Refining**: Use your journal insights to adjust your herbal routines and choices, refining them to better meet your health goals.

Step 12: Continual Learning and Adaptation

The world of herbal medicine is vast. Continual learning and adaptation are key to fully harnessing the benefits of herbs.

1. **Educational Resources**: Utilize books, online courses, workshops, and seminars to expand your knowledge of herbal medicine.

2. **Staying Updated**: Keep abreast of the latest research and developments in the field of herbalism to refine your practices and choices.

Step 13: Seeking Professional Guidance When Necessary

Consult with herbalists or healthcare providers for personalized advice, especially for specific health conditions or when using potent herbs.

1. **Professional Consultations**: Seek advice for developing a personalized herbal regimen, especially if you are dealing with specific health issues or taking medications.

2. **Safety First**: Always prioritize safety, especially when integrating herbs with other medications or treatments.

By following these steps, individuals can create a holistic herbal routine that not only addresses specific health needs but also contributes to a broader sense of well-being. This is not just about the physical benefits of herbs; it's also about fostering a deeper connection with nature and embracing a lifestyle that prioritizes natural, preventive healthcare. By this, individuals embark on a path of natural wellness that is enriching, sustainable, and deeply aligned with the body's innate healing capabilities.

CHAPTER 13: SUSTAINABLE AND ETHICAL SOURCING OF HERBS

In an era where the global demand for herbal products is steadily rising, the sustainable and ethical sourcing of herbs has become a topic of paramount importance. By opening up various aspects of sustainable and ethical sourcing, from cultivation and harvesting to fair trade and ecological considerations, this chapter aims to guide readers through the complexities of responsibly procuring herbs in a way that is both environmentally sound and socially equitable.

The Importance of Sustainable Sourcing

Sustainable sourcing of herbs is crucial to ensure the long-term viability of medicinal plants and the ecosystems in which they thrive.

1. **Preservation of Biodiversity**: Many herbs are harvested from the wild, and unsustainable practices can lead to the depletion of native populations and loss of biodiversity. Sustainable sourcing ensures that these plants can regenerate and that their habitats are preserved.

2. **Impact on Local Ecosystems**: Responsible sourcing practices consider the broader ecological impact of herb cultivation and harvesting, including soil health, water use, and the well-being of local wildlife.

Ethical Considerations in Herbal Sourcing

Ethical sourcing extends beyond environmental concerns, encompassing the fair treatment of workers and respect for indigenous knowledge.

1. **Fair Labor Practices**: Ethical sourcing ensures that workers involved in the cultivation, harvesting, and processing of herbs are paid fair wages and work under safe conditions.

2. **Respecting Indigenous Rights**: Many medicinal herbs are tied to indigenous cultures and traditions. Ethical sourcing involves respecting these cultural connections and ensuring that indigenous communities are fairly compensated and not exploited.

Organic and Biodynamic Farming Practices

Organic and biodynamic farming practices play a significant role in sustainable and ethical herb cultivation.

1. **Organic Farming**: This approach avoids the use of synthetic pesticides and fertilizers, focusing instead on natural methods to maintain soil health and control pests, which is crucial for the sustainability of herb cultivation.

2. **Biodynamic Farming**: Biodynamic agriculture goes a step further, viewing the farm as a cohesive ecosystem and integrating cosmic rhythms and holistic principles into farming practices.

Wildcrafting: Sustainable Harvesting from the Wild

Wildcrafting is the practice of harvesting herbs directly from their natural habitats, and it requires careful management to be sustainable.

1. **Responsible Wildcrafting Practices**: These include harvesting herbs in a way that allows the plant population to regenerate, avoiding overharvesting, and ensuring that the ecological balance of the habitat is maintained.

2. **Legal and Ethical Considerations**: Wildcrafting must also adhere to legal regulations and ethical guidelines, ensuring that wild herb populations are protected and conserved.

The Role of Certifications in Verifying Sustainability

Certifications can play a critical role in ensuring the sustainability and ethical standards of herb sourcing.

1. **Organic Certification**: This verifies that herbs are grown without synthetic pesticides and fertilizers, in a way that supports ecological balance.

2. **Fair Trade Certification**: Fair trade certifications ensure that herbs are sourced under conditions that uphold social and economic equity for workers.

Traceability and Transparency in Herb Sourcing

Traceability and transparency are key to ensuring that herbs are sustainably and ethically sourced.

1. **Tracking the Supply Chain**: Knowing where and how herbs are sourced, right from the farm to the final product, is crucial in ensuring sustainability and ethical practices.

2. **Consumer Awareness**: Educated consumers can make informed decisions and support brands and products that adhere to sustainable and ethical sourcing practices, thereby encouraging a broader shift in the industry.

Sustainable Sourcing and Local Communities

Sustainable sourcing practices often support local communities, both economically and socially.

1. **Community-Based Projects**: Many sustainable herb sourcing initiatives involve working directly with local communities, providing them with fair employment opportunities and supporting community development projects.

2. **Preserving Traditional Knowledge**: These practices often involve learning from and preserving the traditional knowledge of local communities regarding herb cultivation and use.

Challenges in Sustainable and Ethical Sourcing

Despite the growing awareness, there are several challenges in implementing sustainable and ethical sourcing practices.

1. **Global Demand and Supply Pressures**: The increasing global demand for herbal products can put pressure on supply chains, potentially leading to unsustainable and unethical practices.

2. **Complexities of Certification and Regulation**: Navigating the complex world of certifications and regulations can be challenging for suppliers, especially small-scale farmers or wildcrafters.

Technological Advances in Sustainable Herb Sourcing

Technology is playing an increasingly significant role in promoting sustainable herb sourcing.

1. **Agricultural Innovations**: Technological advancements in agriculture, such as precision farming and water-efficient systems, are aiding in more sustainable cultivation practices.

2. **Blockchain for Traceability**: Blockchain technology is being used to enhance the traceability of herbs, allowing

consumers to track the journey of a product from source to shelf.

Education and Consumer Advocacy

Educating consumers and advocating for sustainable and ethical practices is crucial for long-term change.

1. **Awareness Campaigns**: Raising awareness about the importance of sustainable and ethical sourcing among consumers can drive demand for responsibly sourced products.

2. **Advocacy for Policy Change**: Advocacy for stronger policies and regulations around the sourcing of medicinal herbs can lead to more widespread adoption of sustainable practices.

Promoting Local and Seasonal Herb Use

Encouraging the use of locally grown and seasonal herbs can reduce the environmental impact associated with long-distance transportation and promote sustainability.

1. **Supporting Local Herb Growers**: Purchasing herbs from local growers reduces carbon footprint and supports the local economy.

2. **Adapting to Seasonal Availability**: Using herbs that are in season locally can also contribute to sustainability and offer a deeper connection to the natural rhythms of the environment.

Building Sustainable and Ethical Partnerships

Forging partnerships between herb suppliers, businesses, and consumers based on shared values of sustainability and ethics can amplify the impact of these practices.

1. **Collaborations for Change**: Collaborative efforts between various stakeholders can lead to innovative solutions and greater impact in promoting sustainable and ethical herb sourcing.

2. **Shared Responsibility Model**: Embracing a model where all parties involved take responsibility for sustainable practices can lead to more holistic and effective outcomes.

Sustainable and ethical sourcing of herbs is not just an environmental or social issue; it is deeply intertwined with the principles of holistic health and wellness. This chapter invites readers to be part of a movement that values the integrity of the earth and its resources, ensuring that the healing gifts of herbs can be enjoyed for generations to come. Through education, awareness, and action, we can contribute to a more sustainable, ethical, and healthful future, where the relationship between humans and the natural world is nurtured and honored.

GUIDELINES FOR SOURCING HERBS SUSTAINABLY AND ETHICALLY

Sourcing herbs sustainably and ethically is not just a practice but a philosophy that resonates deeply with the respect for nature. It involves a comprehensive approach that considers the ecological footprint, the socio-economic impact on communities involved in herb cultivation and harvesting, and the long-term viability of plant species. This subchapter presents detailed guidelines to ensure that the procurement of herbs aligns with the principles of sustainability and ethics. The focus here is on creating a harmonious balance between benefiting from nature's bounty and preserving its integrity, ensuring that the use of herbal remedies contributes to the health of both individuals and the planet.

Understanding Sustainable Herb Sourcing

Sustainable sourcing involves practices that ensure the long-term health and availability of herb populations and their natural habitats.

1. **Eco-friendly Cultivation Practices**: Choose herbs grown using eco-friendly methods, such as organic farming, which avoids the use of harmful pesticides and fertilizers that can damage the environment.

2. **Wild Harvesting with Care**: If herbs are wild harvested, it's crucial that they are gathered in ways that do not deplete wild stocks. This includes practices like seed scattering and harvesting in a manner that allows the plant to regenerate.

Ethical Considerations in Sourcing Herbs

Ethical sourcing focuses on the human and social aspects of herb production, ensuring fair treatment and compensation for all workers.

1. **Fair Labor Practices**: Support suppliers who implement fair labor practices, providing fair wages and safe working conditions to their workers.

2. **Community Engagement and Support**: Ethical sourcing also involves supporting local communities, particularly in regions where traditional knowledge plays a significant role in herb cultivation and use.

Quality and Purity of Herbs

The quality and purity of herbs are essential not only for their medicinal value but also as indicators of sustainable and ethical sourcing.

1. **Certified Organic Herbs**: Opt for herbs that are certified organic, as this is often a reliable indicator of sustainable farming practices.

2. **Testing for Contaminants**: Ensure that herbs are tested for contaminants like heavy metals, pesticides, and microbes, which can be harmful to health.

Sourcing from Reputable Suppliers

Building relationships with reputable suppliers is key in ensuring the sustainability and ethics of herb sourcing.

1. **Research Suppliers**: Take the time to research suppliers' practices and policies regarding sustainability and ethics. This can include looking into their sourcing methods, certifications, and company ethos.

2. **Transparency**: Choose suppliers who are transparent about their sourcing locations, methods, and the steps they take to ensure sustainability and ethical practices.

Conservation of Endangered Species

Certain herbs are classified as endangered or threatened due to overharvesting and habitat loss.

1. **Avoiding Endangered Herbs**: Be aware of and avoid using herbs that are on endangered lists unless they are cultivated in a manner that does not harm wild populations.

2. **Supporting Conservation Efforts**: Support conservation efforts by choosing suppliers who actively participate in or contribute to the conservation of endangered species and their habitats.

Sustainable Packaging and Shipping

The sustainability of herb sourcing extends to packaging and shipping practices.

1. **Eco-friendly Packaging**: Look for suppliers who use biodegradable, recyclable, or minimal packaging to reduce environmental impact.

2. **Reducing Carbon Footprint in Shipping**: Prefer suppliers who adopt environmentally friendly shipping practices, such as carbon-neutral shipping or bulk shipping options to minimize carbon emissions.

Promoting Biodiversity in Herb Cultivation

Biodiversity in herb cultivation is essential for maintaining ecological balance and ensuring the health of herb populations.

1. **Diverse Crop Cultivation**: Support suppliers who practice crop diversity, which helps in maintaining soil health, controlling pests naturally, and preserving a wide range of plant species.

2. **Permaculture and Agroforestry Practices**: These sustainable agricultural practices mimic natural ecosystems, promoting biodiversity and ecological harmony.

Consumer Responsibility and Education

As consumers, educating ourselves and making informed decisions are crucial steps in supporting sustainable and ethical herb sourcing.

1. **Continuous Learning**: Stay informed about issues related to herb sourcing, including environmental concerns, ethical dilemmas, and new sustainability initiatives.

2. **Making Informed Choices**: Use your purchasing power to support businesses and suppliers who align with sustainable and ethical practices, and encourage others to do the same.

Sustainable and ethical sourcing of herbs is an endeavor that encompasses environmental stewardship, social responsibility, and respect for traditional knowledge. By adhering to the guidelines outlined in this chapter, individuals can contribute to a more sustainable and equitable system of herb production and consumption.

SUPPORTING LOCAL HERBAL COMMUNITIES AND CONSIDERING ENVIRONMENTAL IMPACTS

The ethos of supporting local herbal communities and considering environmental impacts in the sourcing and use of herbs is a cornerstone of sustainable and ethical herbalism. This does not only foster the preservation and propagation of medicinal plants but also supports the livelihoods of local growers and communities, reinforcing the symbiotic relationship between humans and nature. The guidance offered here emphasizes the interconnectedness of health, community well-being, and environmental stewardship.

Engaging with Local Herbalists and Growers

Building relationships with local herbalists and growers can provide access to high-quality, fresh herbs while supporting the local economy.

1. **Purchasing Locally Grown Herbs**: Buying herbs directly from local farmers or herbalists ensures freshness and supports local agriculture.

2. **Participating in Community Herbal Events**: Engaging in local herbal fairs, markets, and workshops can foster community connections and enhance one's understanding of herbs.

Advocating for Ethical Wildcrafting

Ethical wildcrafting ensures that wild herbs are harvested sustainably, protecting them from overexploitation and preserving their natural habitats.

1. **Responsible Harvesting Practices**: Supporting harvesters who adhere to ethical wildcrafting guidelines, such as taking only what is needed and leaving enough for regeneration, is essential.

2. **Educating About Sustainable Foraging**: Providing education on sustainable foraging practices can help protect wild herb populations and their ecosystems.

Supporting Fair Trade and Ethical Business Practices

Fair trade practices ensure that local growers and harvesters are compensated fairly, promoting economic sustainability and social justice.

1. **Choosing Fair Trade Products**: Opting for herbs and herbal products that are certified fair trade supports ethical business practices.

2. **Transparency in Sourcing**: Supporting businesses that provide transparency in their sourcing and supply chain practices helps consumers make informed choices.

Fostering Community-Based Herbal Projects
Community-based projects can empower local communities, preserve traditional knowledge, and promote sustainable practices.

1. **Community Gardens and Herbal Co-ops**: Establishing community herb gardens or cooperatives can provide access to medicinal plants while fostering community involvement and education.

2. **Conservation and Restoration Projects**: Participating in or supporting local conservation and restoration projects for medicinal plants can help maintain biodiversity and ecological health.

Implementing Sustainable Packaging and Distribution
Choosing sustainable packaging and distribution methods reduces the environmental footprint of herbal products.

1. **Eco-friendly Packaging Solutions**: Encouraging the use of biodegradable, recyclable, or reusable packaging for herbal products supports environmental sustainability.

2. **Reducing Carbon Footprint in Distribution**: Opting for local distribution channels or bulk purchasing can minimize transportation emissions associated with the distribution of herbal products.

Promoting Local Herbal Traditions and Culture
Promoting and preserving local herbal traditions and cultures is crucial for maintaining the diversity and richness of herbal knowledge.

1. **Cultural Events and Festivals**: Participating in or organizing cultural events that celebrate local herbal traditions can help preserve and disseminate this knowledge.

2. **Documentation and Research**: Documenting local herbal practices, remedies, and stories contributes to the preservation of this valuable knowledge for future generations.

Advocating for Policy and Regulatory Support
Advocating for supportive policies and regulations is essential for the sustainable development of the herbal sector.

1. **Lobbying for Supportive Legislation**: Engaging in advocacy efforts to lobby for legislation that supports sustainable and ethical herbal practices, such as organic certification, fair trade, and conservation policies.

2. **Participation in Regulatory Processes**: Participating in regulatory processes to ensure that policies and regulations are informed by the needs and perspectives of the local herbal community.

Supporting local herbal communities and considering environmental impacts in herb sourcing encompasses environmental stewardship, social responsibility, cultural preservation, and economic sustainability. Through collective efforts and shared responsibility, we can ensure that the benefits derived from herbal resources are sustainable, equitable, and beneficial for all stakeholders, including future generations.

DISCUSSION AND REFLECTION ON THE IMPORTANCE OF SUSTAINABILITY IN HERBAL PRACTICE

Sustainability in herbal encompasses a broad spectrum of practices, from the cultivation and harvesting of herbs to their processing and distribution. This subchapter opens a discussion and reflection on the critical importance of sustainability in herbal practice, underscoring how it aligns with the ethics of natural medicine and the broader context of environmental stewardship and social responsibility. The focus here is to foster a deeper understanding and commitment among practitioners, consumers, and enthusiasts towards sustainable practices in the field of herbal medicine.

The Ethical Imperative of Sustainability

Sustainability in herbal practice is deeply rooted in ethical considerations. The way we source, use, and promote herbs has significant ethical implications.

1. **Respect for Nature**: Sustainable herbalism is based on a deep respect for nature and an understanding that our health is intrinsically linked to the health of the planet. It recognizes that we must take only what we need and give back to the earth in equal measure.

2. **Ethical Stewardship**: Practitioners of herbal medicine bear a responsibility to steward plant resources wisely, ensuring their availability for future generations.

Sustainable Practices in Personal and Clinical Herbal Use

Sustainability should be integrated into both personal and clinical herbal practices, making it a part of the holistic health ethos.

1. **Mindful Usage**: This involves being mindful of the quantities of herbs used, reducing waste, and considering the ecological and social footprint of each herb or herbal product.

2. **Educating Clients and Patients**: As practitioners, it's essential to educate clients and patients about sustainable herbal practices, encouraging them to make informed choices.

Sustainable Sourcing and Its Challenges

While the intent to source herbs sustainably is commendable, it often comes with challenges that need addressing.

1. **Navigating Certification and Standards**: Understanding and navigating various certifications and standards for sustainable sourcing can be complex.

2. **Balancing Cost and Accessibility**: Often, sustainably sourced herbs can be more costly, posing challenges in making herbal medicine accessible to a broader population.

Reflecting on the Global Impact of Local Practices

The practice of herbal medicine at a local level has a global impact. Reflecting on this interconnectedness is crucial for understanding the role of sustainability.

1. **Understanding the Global Herbal Market**: Recognizing how local practices contribute to global supply chains can foster a deeper understanding of the importance of sustainable practices.

2. **Responsibility to Global Communities**: Herbal practitioners and consumers have a responsibility to consider how their choices affect communities and environments worldwide.

The Role of Community in Sustainable Herbalism

Building and participating in communities focused on sustainable herbalism can amplify efforts and foster collective action.

1. **Community Gardens and Cooperatives**: Engaging in or supporting community gardens and cooperatives can promote sustainable cultivation and sharing of herbal knowledge.

2. **Networks and Alliances**: Forming networks and alliances with other herbalists, growers, and environmental groups can strengthen efforts towards sustainability.

Sustainable Herbalism as an Ethos

Sustainable herbalism is more than a set of practices; it's an ethos that encompasses respect for nature, social responsibility, and a commitment to the health of future generations.

1. **Living the Principles**: Practitioners of sustainable herbalism embody the principles in their personal and professional lives, serving as examples for others.

2. **Commitment to Continuous Learning**: Engaging in continuous learning and adaptation is essential to stay abreast of best practices in sustainable herbalism.

Sustainability in herbal practice is a multi-dimensional concept that extends beyond environmental conservation to encompass social equity, economic viability, and ethical responsibility. As practitioners, consumers, and advocates of herbal medicine, understanding and implementing sustainable practices is imperative to ensure the longevity and efficacy of herbal remedies while protecting the planet and supporting communities.

CHAPTER 14: HERBAL PRESERVATION AND STORAGE

In herbal medicine, the preservation and storage of herbs are as crucial as their cultivation and sourcing. The process of preserving and storing herbs involves understanding the unique properties of each herb and employing methods that best retain their medicinal qualities. This chapter aims to guide enthusiasts, practitioners, and consumers of herbal medicine through various techniques and considerations for effective preservation and storage. By doing so, it ensures that the integrity and healing power of herbs are maintained from harvest to use, aligning with the holistic approach of maximizing therapeutic benefits while minimizing waste and loss of quality.

The Importance of Proper Preservation and Storage

The significance of preserving and storing herbs correctly cannot be overstated. It is a critical step in maintaining the therapeutic properties of herbs.

1. **Retention of Medicinal Properties**: Proper preservation techniques ensure that the active constituents of herbs are retained, thereby guaranteeing their effectiveness when used for medicinal purposes.

2. **Preventing Degradation and Spoilage**: Improper storage can lead to degradation of herbs due to factors like moisture, light, and temperature, resulting in spoilage and loss of medicinal qualities.

Understanding the Basics of Herbal Preservation

Herbal preservation involves a variety of techniques, each suited to different types of herbs and their specific properties.

1. **Drying**: Drying is one of the most common methods of preserving herbs. It involves removing moisture from the herbs, thereby inhibiting the growth of microorganisms that cause decay.

2. **Freezing**: Freezing is another effective method, especially for preserving the flavor and medicinal properties of fresh herbs.

Factors Influencing Herbal Preservation

Several factors influence the effectiveness of herbal preservation, and understanding these is key to choosing the right method.

1. **Moisture Content**: Herbs with high moisture content, like basil or mint, may require different preservation techniques compared to those with lower moisture content.

2. **Herb Type and Form**: The preservation method may vary depending on whether the herb is a leaf, flower, root, or seed.

Storing Preserved Herbs

Once preserved, proper storage of herbs is crucial to maintaining their quality over time.

1. **Airtight Containers**: Herbs should be stored in airtight containers to protect them from moisture and air, which can lead to spoilage.

2. **Cool, Dark, and Dry Storage**: Herbs are best stored in cool, dark, and dry places to prevent degradation from light and heat.

Labeling and Organization

Proper labeling and organization of stored herbs are important for ease of use and maintaining effectiveness.

1. **Labeling with Date and Name**: Each container of preserved herbs should be labeled with the herb's name and the date of preservation to track freshness and potency.

2. **Organized Storage System**: Organizing herbs systematically, perhaps alphabetically or by type, can facilitate easy access and ensure that older herbs are used first.

Long-term Storage Considerations

For long-term storage, special considerations are necessary to ensure herbs remain effective and safe for use.

1. **Vacuum Sealing**: Vacuum sealing can be an effective method for long-term storage, especially for herbs that are susceptible to moisture and air exposure.

2. **Monitoring for Quality**: Regularly checking stored herbs for signs of spoilage or loss of potency is important, especially for herbs stored over extended periods.

Special Techniques for Specific Herbs

Certain herbs may require special preservation techniques due to their unique properties.

1. **Preserving Volatile Oils**: Herbs with volatile oils, such as peppermint or eucalyptus, may require quick drying or freezing methods to retain their essential oils.

2. **Storing Roots and Barks**: Roots and barks often require different preservation techniques, such as slicing and drying at specific temperatures, to ensure their medicinal constituents are maintained.

Impact of Preservation on Herbal Efficacy

The method of preservation can impact the efficacy of herbs, making it crucial to choose methods that align with the intended use of the herb.

1. **Retention of Active Constituents**: Preservation methods should be chosen based on their ability to retain the active constituents relevant to the herb's medicinal use.

2. **Considerations for Therapeutic Use**: The intended therapeutic use of the herb should guide the choice of preservation method to ensure maximum efficacy.

Sustainable and Ethical Considerations in Preservation

Sustainability and ethics should also guide the preservation and storage of herbs, reflecting a holistic approach to herbalism.

1. **Environmentally Friendly Methods**: Preference should be given to preservation methods that have a minimal environmental impact, such as air drying or using energy-efficient dehydrators.

2. **Ethical Sourcing and Preservation**: Ethical considerations should extend to preservation, ensuring that the methods used

do not negatively impact the environment or local communities.

Innovations in Herbal Preservation

Technological innovations are continually offering new methods for herbal preservation that can enhance efficacy and convenience.

1. **Advanced Dehydration Techniques**: New dehydration technologies can preserve herbs more efficiently, retaining a higher level of their medicinal properties.

2. **Preservation for Commercial Use**: Innovations in preservation are particularly important for commercial herbal products, ensuring consistency, safety, and efficacy on a large scale.

The preservation and storage of herbs are critical components of herbal medicine, ensuring that the healing powers of herbs are available when needed. Proper preservation and storage not only extend the life of herbs but also uphold the principles of sustainability and ethical practice in herbalism. This chapter provides a comprehensive guide to preserving and storing herbs, offering practical solutions for both home herbalists and professional practitioners.

TECHNIQUES FOR PRESERVING AND STORING HERBS

The preservation and storage of herbs is critical for maintaining the herbs' medicinal properties and ensuring their longevity. These techniques are not just about prolonging the shelf life of herbs but are deeply intertwined with the philosophy of maximizing their therapeutic benefits. This subchapter reiterates various methods and techniques for preserving and storing herbs. It offers detailed insights into the best practices that ensure herbs retain their potency, flavor, and healing properties over time.

Drying Herbs

Drying is one of the most traditional and effective methods for preserving herbs. It involves removing moisture from the herbs, which prevents the growth of bacteria and mold.

1. **Air Drying**: This is a simple and natural method, suitable for most herbs, especially leafy ones like basil, oregano, and mint. Herbs are tied in small bundles and hung upside down in a warm, dry, and well-ventilated area away from direct sunlight.

2. **Oven Drying**: For quicker drying, herbs can be placed on a baking sheet in a low-temperature oven. This method requires careful monitoring to prevent burning and ensure even drying.

3. **Using Dehydrators**: Dehydrators are ideal for controlling temperature and air flow, making them suitable for drying a variety of herbs. They are particularly useful in humid climates where air drying is less effective.

Freezing Herbs

Freezing preserves the flavor and some of the medicinal properties of herbs, particularly those with high moisture content.

1. **Freezing in Water**: Herbs can be chopped and frozen in ice cube trays with water. This method is great for herbs used in cooking, as the cubes can be directly added to dishes.

2. **Freezing in Oil**: Herbs can also be frozen in oil, which is ideal for herbs used in sautéing and frying. The oil helps preserve the flavor and texture of the herbs.

3. **Blanching Before Freezing**: For some herbs, blanching before freezing can help retain color and flavor. This involves briefly boiling the herbs and then plunging them into ice water before freezing.

Creating Herbal Infused Oils

Infused oils are another way to preserve the medicinal properties of herbs, especially those with volatile oils.

1. **Cold Infusion Method**: Herbs are soaked in oil, such as olive or almond oil, for several weeks in a warm, sunny spot, then strained and stored.

2. **Heat Infusion Method**: For a quicker process, herbs and oil can be gently heated over a double boiler for a few hours, then strained and stored.

Preserving Herbs in Vinegar and Honey

Vinegar and Honey are also effective mediums for preserving certain herbs.

1. **Herbal Vinegars**: Herbs can be steeped in vinegar to create flavorful and medicinal preparations. Apple cider vinegar is commonly used due to its own health benefits.

2. **Herbal Honeys**: Soaking herbs in Honey not only preserves their properties but also creates a pleasant medicinal product. This is particularly useful for herbs used in soothing sore throats and coughs.

Long-term Preservation Strategies

For long-term storage, some additional strategies can be employed.

1. **Vacuum Sealing**: Vacuum-sealed bags can extend the shelf life of dried herbs by protecting them from air and moisture.

2. **Silica Gel Packs**: Including silica gel packs in herb containers can help absorb any excess moisture and keep the herbs dry.

Quality Checks and Routine Monitoring

Regular monitoring is key to ensuring the herbs maintain their quality over time.

1. **Periodic Quality Checks**: Regularly check stored herbs for any signs of degradation, such as changes in color, smell, or texture.

2. **Rotating Stock**: Use a first-in, first-out system to ensure older stocks are used before newer ones, maintaining the freshness and potency of the herbs.

Sustainable Practices in Preservation and Storage
Sustainability should also be considered in the preservation and storage of herbs.

1. **Eco-friendly Packaging**: Opt for environmentally friendly packaging materials, such as glass or recyclable plastics.

2. **Energy Efficiency**: When using methods like dehydrating or freezing, consider the energy efficiency of appliances to minimize the environmental impact.

Effective preservation and storage of herbs are foundational to the practice of herbal medicine, ensuring that the full therapeutic potential of herbs is available when needed. By understanding and applying the various techniques of drying, freezing, tincturing, and oil infusion, as well as proper storage methods, practitioners and enthusiasts can ensure the longevity and efficacy of their herbal remedies.

PRACTICAL TIPS AND 'HOMEWORK' FOR IMPLEMENTING EFFECTIVE PRESERVATION TECHNIQUES

Implementing effective preservation techniques for herbs requires more than just an understanding of various methods; it demands practical application and consistent practice. This subchapter is dedicated to providing hands-on tips and actionable 'homework' assignments for individuals looking to integrate effective herb preservation techniques into their routine. These practical exercises are designed to deepen one's skills and knowledge in herbal preservation, ensuring that the medicinal properties of herbs are maintained for their optimal use.

Practical Tip 1: Establishing a Drying Routine

A consistent drying routine is fundamental for preserving many types of herbs.

Homework Assignment:

- Identify three commonly used herbs in your kitchen or herbal practice.

- Research the optimal drying method for each herb (air drying, oven drying, dehydrating).

- Practice drying each herb using the identified method and document the process, including time taken and changes observed in the herbs.

Practical Tip 2: Creating Your Own Herbal Tinctures

Making herbal tinctures is an excellent way to preserve herbs' medicinal properties.

Homework Assignment:

- Follow a step-by-step guide to create your tincture, label it with the date and contents, and monitor the tincture over a four to six-week period, shaking it daily.

Practical Tip 3: Experimenting with Freezing Techniques

Freezing herbs is a quick way to preserve their freshness, especially for culinary use.

Homework Assignment:

- Select two herbs with high moisture content, such as basil or cilantro.

- Experiment with different freezing techniques: freezing in water, oil, and as a pesto or puree.

- Document the flavor and texture of these herbs after thawing and use them in a cooking recipe to evaluate their preserved quality.

Practical Tip 4: Vacuum Sealing Dried Herbs

Vacuum sealing can significantly extend the shelf life of dried herbs.

Homework Assignment:

- After drying a batch of herbs, use a vacuum sealer to package them.

- Store these herbs for a month, then open and evaluate their condition compared to non-vacuum sealed herbs in terms of aroma, texture, and color.

Practical Tip 5: Making and Storing Herbal Infused Oils

Herbal oils are both therapeutic and can be used in cooking.

Homework Assignment:

- Choose a herb and a carrier oil (like olive or almond oil) to create an infused oil.

- Use either the cold infusion method or the heat infusion method to prepare your herbal oil.

- Store the oil in a cool, dark place and use it within a specified time, noting any changes in its properties.

Practical Tip 6: Building a Herbal Storage System

Proper storage is as important as the preservation method itself.

Homework Assignment:

- Designate a storage area in your home that is cool, dark, and dry.

- Organize your preserved herbs, tinctures, and oils in this area using airtight containers, proper labeling, and a first-in, first-out system.

- Regularly check this area for any signs of spoilage or degradation.

Practical Tip 7: Utilizing Natural Antioxidants in Preservation

Natural antioxidants can enhance the shelf life of oil-based herbal preparations.

Homework Assignment:

- Research natural antioxidants such as Vitamin E or rosemary extract.

- Add these antioxidants to one of your herbal oil preparations.

- Compare the shelf life and quality of this preparation with another batch without antioxidants over a period.

Practical Tip 8: Learning Through Observation

Observation is a key aspect of mastering herbal preservation.

Homework Assignment:

- Select several herbs with different preservation needs (such as leafy herbs, roots, and flowers).

- Apply a suitable preservation method to each (drying, freezing, tincturing, etc.) and closely observe and record the changes over time, noting aspects like color, texture, scent, and any signs of spoilage.

Practical Tip 9: Experimenting with Herbal Vinegars and Honeys

Herbal vinegars and Honeys are not only medicinal but also culinary delights.

Homework Assignment:

- Create a herbal vinegar using Apple cider vinegar and a herb of your choice. Let it infuse for 4-6 weeks, shaking it regularly.

- Similarly, prepare a herbal Honey by infusing raw Honey with a different herb.

- Use these preparations in cooking or as a remedy and note their flavors, effectiveness, and shelf life.

Practical Tip 10: Implementing a Rotational System for Herb Use

A rotational system ensures that herbs are used while they are most potent.

Homework Assignment:

- Organize your herbs and herbal preparations according to their preservation dates.

- Plan to use the oldest items first and rotate stock regularly.

- Keep track of the usage and replenishment of your herbs to maintain a fresh and effective supply.

Practical Tip 11: Engaging in Continuous Learning

The field of herbal preservation is ever-evolving, and continuous learning is key.

Homework Assignment:

- Subscribe to herbal journals, join online forums, or participate in workshops focused on herbal preservation.

- Implement at least one new preservation technique you learn every few months.

- Share your learnings and experiences with a community of herbal enthusiasts.

Practical Tip 12: Sustainability in Herbal Preservation

Sustainability should be a guiding principle in your preservation practices.

Homework Assignment:

- Audit your current preservation methods for their environmental impact.

- Research and implement at least one more eco-friendly preservation method, such as using solar dehydrators or recycling jars for tinctures.

- Evaluate the changes and consider their long-term sustainability benefits.

Mastering the art of preserving and storing herbs is a vital skill in herbalism, ensuring that the healing properties of herbs are available whenever needed. Through these practical tips and hands-on homework assignments, individuals can develop a deeper understanding and proficiency in various herbal preservation techniques. As each herb is unique in its preservation needs, the continuous application and refinement of these techniques are essential.

CHAPTER 15: HERBAL FIRST AID KIT

The concept of a herbal first aid kit takes a central stage in health and wellness, offering a natural and effective alternative to conventional first aid methods. This chapter provides an in-depth explanation of creating and utilizing a herbal first aid kit, a vital component for anyone seeking to integrate natural remedies into their healthcare practices. The herbal first aid kit is a testament to the power and versatility of herbs in addressing a wide range of common ailments and emergencies. This comprehensive guide depicts the selection of herbs, preparation of remedies, and practical applications, ensuring that individuals are well-equipped to handle minor health issues with natural, effective solutions.

The Essence of a Herbal First Aid Kit

The essence of a herbal first aid kit lies in its ability to offer immediate, accessible, and natural remedies for various common health concerns.

1. **Natural and Holistic Approach**: A herbal first aid kit embodies the principles of natural medicine, offering remedies that work in harmony with the body's natural healing processes.

2. **Empowerment through Self-Care**: Equipping oneself with a herbal first aid kit is an empowering step towards taking charge of one's health and well-being, reducing reliance on synthetic medications for minor ailments.

Selecting Herbs for the First Aid Kit

The selection of herbs for a first aid kit is a thoughtful process, guided by the herbs' medicinal properties and the types of ailments they can address.

1. **Broad-Spectrum Herbs**: Including herbs with broad-spectrum healing properties, such as calendula for skin issues or chamomile for digestive discomfort, is crucial.

2. **Specific Remedies for Common Ailments**: Herbs like peppermint for headaches, Aloe vera for burns, or echinacea for immune support, are essential in a well-rounded kit.

Preparation of Herbal Remedies

The preparation of herbal remedies is a key aspect of building a first aid kit, involving various forms such as tinctures, salves, oils, and teas.

1. **Tinctures for Longevity**: Preparing tinctures of certain herbs ensures that their medicinal properties are preserved for longer periods and are readily available for use.

2. **Salves and Ointments for Topical Application**: Creating salves and ointments for external use, such as comfrey salve for bruises or Tea tree oil ointment for antiseptic needs.

Practical Applications of Herbal Remedies

Understanding the practical applications of each herb and remedy in the kit is vital for effective first aid.

1. **Knowledge of Herbal Actions**: Familiarity with the actions of herbs, such as anti-inflammatory, antiseptic, or analgesic properties, allows for their appropriate application in various situations.

2. **Method of Application**: Knowing how to apply each remedy, whether it be a poultice, a compress, or an oral administration, is essential for the efficacy of the treatment.

Safety and Precautions

While herbal remedies are generally safe, understanding their proper use and potential contraindications is crucial.

1. **Allergies and Sensitivities**: Being aware of potential allergic reactions or sensitivities to certain herbs and testing them before widespread use.

2. **Interactions with Medications**: Knowledge of any possible interactions between herbal remedies and prescription medications.

Customizing the Herbal First Aid Kit

Customizing the first aid kit to suit individual or family needs ensures that it is tailored to specific health requirements and preferences.

1. **Personalization Based on Lifestyle**: Including remedies that align with one's lifestyle, activities, and common health issues faced.

2. **Family-Specific Needs**: Adjusting the kit to include remedies suitable for children or elderly family members, considering their specific health needs.

Portability and Accessibility

Designing the first aid kit for portability and ease of access is important, especially for those who travel or spend a lot of time outdoors.

1. **Compact and Travel-Friendly Design**: Organizing the kit in a compact, portable container that can easily fit in a backpack or car.

2. **Labeling and Organization**: Clearly labeling each remedy and organizing the kit in a way that makes it easy to find what is needed quickly in an emergency.

Education and Training

Possessing the knowledge and skills to use the herbal first aid kit effectively is as crucial as the kit itself.

1. **Learning Herbal First Aid Techniques**: Acquiring knowledge through books, courses, or workshops on how to use each herb and remedy in the kit.

2. **Practice and Familiarization**: Regularly practicing the preparation and application of remedies to become comfortable and efficient in using the kit.

Sustainable and Ethical Sourcing of Herbs

Ensuring that the herbs and ingredients in the first aid kit are sourced sustainably and ethically aligns with the principles of holistic health.

1. **Choosing Ethically Sourced Herbs**: Opting for herbs that are grown and harvested sustainably, respecting environmental and social ethics.

2. **Supporting Local Herb Suppliers**: Where possible, sourcing herbs from local growers or suppliers to support community businesses and reduce the ecological footprint.

Regular Maintenance of the Kit

Regular maintenance of the herbal first aid kit ensures that its contents remain effective and safe to use.

1. **Checking Expiry Dates**: Regularly checking and replacing any remedies that have expired or lost their potency.

2. **Restocking and Updating**: Keeping the kit stocked and updating it with new remedies or herbs as needed.

Incorporating Complementary Tools and Supplies

In addition to herbal remedies, incorporating other complementary tools and supplies can enhance the functionality of the first aid kit.

1. **Essential Tools**: Including items such as scissors, tweezers, cotton swabs, and bandages to assist in the application of remedies.

2. **Educational Materials**: Carrying a small guide or notes on the use of each herb and remedy for quick reference.

Addressing a Range of Health Concerns

A well-prepared herbal first aid kit can address a range of health concerns from minor injuries to common ailments.

1. **Minor Injuries**: Including herbs and remedies for cuts, bruises, insect bites, and sprains.

2. **Common Ailments**: Having remedies on hand for issues like indigestion, headaches, stress, or insomnia.

Creating and maintaining a herbal first aid kit is a rewarding endeavor that enhances one's ability to respond to health concerns with natural, effective solutions. The herbal first aid kit is not only a toolkit for wellness but also a symbol of a lifestyle that values and utilizes the healing power of nature, reflecting a deep understanding and respect for the ancient wisdom of herbalism.

BUILDING A BASIC KIT OF HERBAL REMEDIES FOR IMMEDIATE NEEDS

Creating a basic herbal first aid kit involves a thoughtful selection of herbs and natural remedies targeted at addressing immediate and common health concerns. This subchapter searches deeper into the the importance of choosing a range of herbs that are versatile, effective, and safe for various situations, from minor injuries to everyday health complaints.

Essential Herbs for Immediate Needs

Certain herbs are particularly useful for immediate needs due to their specific healing properties.

1. **Calendula**: Known for its skin-healing properties, calendula is ideal for cuts, scrapes, and mild burns. It can be included in the kit as a cream, ointment, or tincture.

2. **Peppermint**: Useful for digestive issues, headaches, and as a cooling agent, peppermint can be included as tea or oil.

Tools and Supplies for the Herbal Kit

In addition to herbal remedies, certain tools and supplies are essential for a well-equipped first aid kit.

1. **Application Tools**: Include items such as cotton balls, swabs, and small spatulas for applying salves and ointments.

2. **Storage Containers**: Opt for small, durable containers that protect the remedies from light and air, such as amber glass bottles for tinctures and metal tins for salves.

Simple Home Preparations

Some effective first aid remedies can be prepared easily at home, providing a cost-effective and personalized approach to herbal first aid.

1. **Aloe vera Gel**: Fresh Aloe vera gel, extracted from the leaves of the aloe plant, is excellent for burns, sunburn, and skin irritation.

2. **Herbal Teas**: Packets of dried herbs like chamomile or ginger can be included for making teas to address issues like stress or indigestion.

Addressing Common Ailments

The kit should contain remedies that address a variety of common ailments, from skin issues to respiratory problems.

1. **Respiratory Relief**: Herbs like thyme, known for its expectorant properties, or eucalyptus oil for inhalation, can be included for respiratory concerns.

2. **Pain and Fever**: Willow bark, nature's aspirin, can be used for pain relief and fever reduction.

Organizing and Maintaining the Kit

A well-organized and regularly maintained kit is essential for ensuring the remedies are effective when needed.

1. **Organization**: Organize the remedies in a way that makes them easy to find and use. Grouping them by type (such as tinctures, salves, teas) or by the ailment they address can be helpful.

2. **Regular Checks**: Regularly check the contents of the kit for expiration dates, potency, and condition. Replace any items that are past their prime or have been used up.

Educational Components

Including educational materials in the kit can provide valuable information on how to use the remedies effectively.

1. **Herbal First Aid Guide**: Create or include a small guidebook or pamphlet that provides basic information on each herb and remedy in the kit.

2. **Emergency Contacts**: List contacts for emergency medical help and advice, as well as contacts for local herbalists or naturopaths for non-emergency queries.

Building a basic herbal first aid kit is a proactive step towards embracing natural health solutions for common ailments and emergencies. It requires careful selection, preparation, and organization of a variety of herbal remedies, each chosen for its specific healing properties and ease of use. Such a kit reflects a commitment to a holistic and natural approach to health and wellness.

QUICK REFERENCE GUIDE FOR EMERGENCY HERBAL TREATMENTS

In emergency situations, having a quick reference guide for herbal treatments can be invaluable. This subchapter focuses on developing a comprehensive, easy-to-navigate guide that outlines the use of herbal remedies for various emergency scenario. Such a guide is a resource that empowers individuals to respond with confidence and knowledge when faced with health crises, using natural and effective remedies.

Understanding Herbal Emergency Treatments

Before diving into the specific remedies, it's essential to understand the role and scope of herbal treatments in emergencies.

1. **Role of Herbal Remedies in Emergencies**: Herbal remedies can provide immediate relief for various conditions and support the body's natural healing process.

2. **Limitations and When to Seek Medical Help**: Recognize the limitations of herbal remedies and understand when it's crucial to seek professional medical assistance.

Creating the Quick Reference Guide

Developing a guide that is easy to use and understand is key to its effectiveness in emergencies.

1. **Clear Layout and Organization**: Organize the guide by types of emergencies (e.g., cuts, burns, allergic reactions) for quick access.

2. **Simple and Direct Instructions**: Provide clear, concise instructions on how to prepare and use each remedy.

Remedies for Cuts and Wounds

In the case of minor cuts and wounds, certain herbs can play a crucial role in cleaning and aiding the healing process.

1. **Calendula for Healing**: Known for its antiseptic and healing properties, calendula can be applied as a salve or wash.

2. **Yarrow to Stop Bleeding**: Yarrow is effective in stopping bleeding and can be applied directly to the wound.

Herbal Treatments for Allergic Reactions

Allergic reactions can be sudden and uncomfortable, and certain herbs can provide quick relief.

1. **Nettle for Allergies**: Nettle is known to relieve allergic symptoms and can be taken as a tea or tincture.

2. **Chamomile for Skin Reactions**: Chamomile, applied topically as a compress, can soothe skin reactions like hives.

Handling Digestive Emergencies

Digestive emergencies like nausea, indigestion, or diarrhea can be alleviated with specific herbal remedies.

1. **Ginger for Nausea**: Ginger is effective in treating nausea and can be taken as tea or chewed raw.

2. **Peppermint for Indigestion**: Peppermint tea can relieve indigestion and soothe the stomach.

Respiratory Issues and Herbal Solutions

In cases of minor respiratory issues like coughs or congestion, certain herbs can offer relief.

1. **Eucalyptus for Congestion**: Eucalyptus steam inhalation can clear nasal congestion and ease breathing.

2. **Thyme for Coughs**: Thyme has expectorant properties and can be used in a tea to relieve coughs.

Stress and Anxiety Relief

Herbs can play a significant role in managing sudden stress and anxiety.

1. **Lavender for Calming**: Lavender, used in aromatherapy or as a tea, can have a calming effect on the nerves.

2. **Lemon Balm for Anxiety**: Lemon balm, known for its mild sedative properties, can be taken as a tea to alleviate symptoms of anxiety.

Herbal First Aid for Headaches

Headaches, whether tension-related or migraines, can be effectively managed with certain herbs.

1. **Peppermint Oil for Tension Headaches**: Applied topically, peppermint oil can provide relief from tension headaches.

2. **Feverfew for Migraines**: Feverfew is a well-known herb for preventing and treating migraines and can be taken in capsule or tea form.

Dealing with Insomnia and Sleep Issues

Herbs can offer a natural solution for insomnia and other sleep disturbances.

1. **Valerian Root for Insomnia**: Valerian root, known for its sedative qualities, can be taken as a tincture or tea for inducing sleep.

2. **Chamomile for Restless Sleep**: A cup of chamomile tea before bed can promote a restful and peaceful sleep.

Treating Muscle Aches and Pain

For muscle aches and pains, certain herbs can provide soothing relief.

1. **Comfrey for Muscle Pain**: Comfrey, used as a poultice or salve, can relieve muscle pain and speed up healing.

2. **Cayenne Pepper for Topical Pain Relief**: Cayenne pepper, used in a salve, can help reduce muscle soreness and joint pain.

Bites and Stings: Herbal Interventions

Herbal remedies can be effective in treating insect bites and stings.

1. **Plantain for Bites and Stings**: Plantain, applied as a fresh poultice, can reduce itching and swelling from insect bites.

2. **Witch hazel for Inflammation**: Witch hazel can be used as a soothing agent for bites, reducing inflammation and discomfort.

Safety Considerations and Disclaimer

The guide should include safety considerations and a disclaimer, emphasizing the importance of understanding each herb's properties and potential interactions.

1. **Highlight Allergy Warnings**: Include warnings about potential allergic reactions to certain herbs.

2. **Emphasis on Professional Medical Advice**: Remind users to seek professional medical advice for serious or uncertain conditions.

Regular Updates and Review

Keeping the guide updated with the latest information and research ensures its continued relevance and effectiveness.

1. **Annual Review of Contents**: Regularly review and update the guide to include new findings, additional herbs, or revised recommendations.

2. **Feedback and Improvement**: Encourage users to provide feedback on the guide, facilitating continuous improvement and refinement.

A quick reference guide for emergency herbal treatments is an invaluable resource for anyone embracing a holistic approach to health. As users become more familiar with the guide and its contents, they develop greater confidence and skill in utilizing herbal remedies.

CHAPTER 16: EMPOWERING YOURSELF THROUGH HERBAL KNOWLEDGE

In this age of information overload and quick-fix solutions, taking the time to understand and embrace the wisdom of herbal medicine offers a pathway to deeper health insights and a more attuned way of living. This chapter is dedicated to exploring how individuals can empower themselves through the acquisition and application of herbal knowledge. This exploration aims to inspire and equip readers with the tools and confidence to integrate herbal knowledge into their daily lives, fostering a sense of autonomy and connection with the natural world.

The Roots of Herbal Knowledge

Herbal knowledge has ancient origins, deeply intertwined with the evolution of human societies and cultures.

1. **Historical Significance:** Herbalism's roots can be traced back to ancient civilizations, where it was integral to both healing practices and spiritual rituals. This rich history provides a foundation for modern herbal knowledge.

2. **Cultural Diversity in Herbal Practices**: The use of herbs varies widely across cultures, each bringing its unique perspective and practices. Understanding this diversity enriches one's own herbal practice and promotes a deeper respect for different healing traditions.

Understanding Plant Medicine

At the heart of herbal knowledge is an understanding of plants as medicine, in all their complexity and diversity.

1. **Botanical Basics**: A fundamental understanding of plant biology, including plant anatomy and life cycles, lays the groundwork for recognizing and utilizing medicinal plants effectively.

2. **Phytochemistry and Herbal Constituents**: Knowledge of the active chemical constituents in plants and how they interact with the human body is crucial for using herbs safely and effectively.

Personal Empowerment through Herbal Education

Empowering oneself through herbal education involves a proactive approach to learning and applying herbal knowledge.

1. **Self-Study and Research**: Engaging in self-study, such as reading herbal texts, attending workshops, or participating in online courses, allows individuals to build a solid foundation of herbal knowledge.

2. **Practical Application**: Applying what is learned through personal experimentation and practice, such as making herbal remedies or growing medicinal plants, reinforces knowledge and builds confidence.

Building a Herbal Home Pharmacy

Creating a home pharmacy with a collection of essential herbs and herbal preparations empowers individuals to manage common health issues naturally.

1. **Selection of Key Herbs**: Choosing herbs that are versatile and address a range of common ailments allows for a well-rounded home pharmacy.

2. **Preparation and Storage of Herbal Remedies**: Learning to prepare and store herbal remedies, such as tinctures, salves, and teas, ensures they are available when needed.

Herbalism in the Modern World

Understanding the role and relevance of herbalism in today's world, amidst advancements in medicine and technology, is vital for its informed application.

1. **Complementing Conventional Medicine**: Recognizing how herbal medicine can complement conventional medical treatments, offering holistic approaches to health and wellness.

2. **Navigating Legal and Ethical Considerations**: Being aware of the legal and ethical considerations surrounding the use of herbal medicine is crucial, especially regarding claims of efficacy and safety.

Research and Evidence-based Practice

Incorporating research and evidence-based approaches into herbal practice enhances its credibility and effectiveness.

1. **Staying Informed of Current Research**: Keeping abreast of the latest research in herbal medicine, including clinical studies and trials, helps in making informed decisions about herbal use.

2. **Critical Evaluation of Sources**: Learning to critically evaluate the sources of herbal information, distinguishing between anecdotal experiences and scientifically validated data.

Personal Health Autonomy

Empowering oneself with herbal knowledge leads to greater personal health autonomy, allowing individuals to take more control over their health and wellness.

1. **Making Informed Health Choices**: Herbal knowledge enables individuals to make informed choices about their health, exploring natural alternatives where appropriate.

2. **Advocacy for One's Health**: Being knowledgeable about herbs allows individuals to advocate for their health, whether in preventive measures or in seeking complementary treatments.

Empowering oneself through herbal knowledge involves a deep engagement with the natural world, a commitment to sustainable and ethical practices, and a dedication to continual learning and growth. This empowerment through herbal knowledge fosters a greater sense of autonomy, resilience, and harmony with the environment, highlighting the enduring relevance and value of plant medicine in contemporary life.

TOOLS AND RESOURCES FOR CONTINUING EDUCATION IN HERBAL MEDICINE REFLECTING O'NEILL'S COMMITMENT

This subchapter outlines the various tools and resources available for those seeking to deepen their knowledge and practice in herbal medicine. Here, we will launch into a range of educational tools and resources, from traditional methods to modern digital platforms, each offering unique opportunities for growth and learning in the field of herbalism. This guide aims to provide readers with a comprehensive understanding of how to continuously expand their herbal knowledge and skills, aligning with O'Neill's vision of empowering individuals through education and self-awareness in natural health.

Comprehensive Herbal Texts and Books

Building a library of herbal texts is foundational for anyone serious about their education in herbal medicine.

1. **Classic Herbal Medicine Books**: Start with the classics - texts that have stood the test of time and provide a solid foundation in herbal knowledge.

2. **Modern Herbal Publications**: Supplement your library with modern publications that offer the latest research, clinical studies, and contemporary applications of herbal medicine.

Enrolling in Herbal Medicine Courses

Structured courses provide a systematic approach to learning, from basic to advanced levels.

1. **Local Workshops and Classes**: Participate in workshops and classes offered by local herbalists or health centers. These often provide hands-on experience with herbs.

2. **Online Herbal Medicine Courses**: Leverage the flexibility and diversity of online courses, which can range from introductory lessons to specialized topics in herbalism.

Herbal Medicine Schools and Institutes

For those seeking a more formal and comprehensive education, attending a school or institute dedicated to herbal medicine is a significant step.

1. **Accredited Herbal Programs**: Research and consider enrolling in accredited programs that offer certifications or degrees in herbal medicine.

2. **Specialized Training**: Some institutions offer specialized training in areas like ethnobotany, herbal pharmacology, or clinical herbalism.

Utilizing Digital Platforms and Resources

The digital age has opened up a wealth of resources for herbal education.

1. **Online Forums and Communities**: Engage with online forums and communities where herbalists, both novice and experienced, share insights, ask questions, and offer advice.

2. **Webinars and Online Lectures**: Attend webinars and online lectures hosted by experts in the field. These can provide up-to-date information and new perspectives on various herbal topics.

Field Work and Botanical Studies

Practical experience is invaluable in herbal education. Engaging in field work and botanical studies deepens understanding and appreciation for plants.

1. **Herb Walks and Botanical Tours**: Participate in guided herb walks or botanical tours to learn about plant identification, habitats, and traditional uses.

2. **Botanical Gardens and Herbariums**: Visit botanical gardens and herbariums to study a wide variety of plants and their characteristics.

Mentorship and Apprenticeships
Learning under the guidance of an experienced herbalist through mentorship or apprenticeships can be profoundly impactful.

1. **Seeking a Mentor**: Connect with an experienced herbalist who can provide personalized guidance, share practical wisdom, and offer insights from their own journey.

2. **Apprenticeship Programs**: Consider apprenticeship programs that offer immersive learning experiences, from harvesting herbs to preparing remedies and understanding their application.

Herbal Conferences and Symposia

Attending conferences and symposia is a great way to stay abreast of the latest developments in herbal medicine and network with professionals in the field.

1. **National and International Conferences**: Attend conferences that bring together herbalists, healthcare professionals, researchers, and educators from around the world.

2. **Specialized Symposia**: Look out for symposia focusing on specific areas of herbal medicine, such as women's health, herbal pharmacology, or integrative medicine practices.

Developing a Personal Herbal Practice

Developing a personal herbal practice is a dynamic way to apply and test one's knowledge.

1. **Personal Herb Garden**: Cultivating a personal herb garden allows for hands-on experience in growing, harvesting, and using herbs.

2. **DIY Herbal Preparations**: Experiment with making your own herbal preparations such as tinctures, salves, and teas. This hands-on practice reinforces learning and builds practical skills.

Self-Study and Independent Research

Self-motivated study and research are crucial for deepening one's understanding of herbal medicine.

1. **Independent Research Projects**: Undertake independent research projects on specific herbs, their uses, or herbal medicine practices.

2. **Staying Informed on Scientific Research**: Regularly read scientific journals and articles related to herbal medicine to stay informed about new findings and perspectives.

Integrating Technology in Herbal Learning

Utilizing technology can enhance the learning experience and provide access to a wide range of resources.

1. **Herbal Medicine Apps**: Use apps related to herbal medicine for quick reference, plant identification, or dosage calculations.

2. **Online Research Databases**: Access online databases and libraries for scholarly articles and research papers on herbal medicine.

Empowering oneself through continuous education in herbal medicine offers profound insights into health, healing, and the natural world. This contributes to the broader community by preserving and spreading the invaluable knowledge of herbal medicine.

EXPERIMENTATION AND ADAPTATION OF HERBAL RECIPES

In the landscape of herbal medicine, experimentation and adaptation stand as pillars of personal and communal growth in the field. This subchapter reports the art and science of tailoring herbal recipes, exploring how personal experimentation and creative adaptation can lead to more effective, personalized herbal remedies. Here, we will uncover the processes and considerations involved in modifying traditional herbal recipes, fostering an innovative spirit that aligns with O'Neill's philosophy of practical, experiential learning.

The Foundation of Herbal Experimentation

Experimentation in herbal medicine is grounded in understanding the fundamental principles of how herbs work.

1. **Understanding Herbal Properties**: A deep understanding of individual herbs, their properties, actions, and potential interactions is crucial for safe and effective experimentation.

2. **Traditional vs. Contemporary Contexts**: Recognizing how traditional herbal recipes can be adapted to contemporary contexts, including modern lifestyles and health challenges.

Developing Intuition and Observation Skills

Intuition, backed by observation and experience, plays a significant role in herbal experimentation.

1. **Intuitive Blending of Herbs**: Developing an intuitive sense for which herbs to combine, guided by an understanding of their synergistic effects.

2. **Observational Learning**: Paying close attention to the effects of herbal remedies, and using these observations to refine and improve recipes.

The Role of Personal Health Experiences

Personal health experiences often serve as a catalyst for herbal experimentation.

1. **Learning from Personal Health Journeys**: Using one's own or close ones' health experiences as a basis for experimenting with herbal remedies.

2. **Adapting Recipes for Personal Health Needs**: Modifying traditional recipes to better suit personal health conditions or goals.

Feedback Loops and Continuous Improvement

Creating a feedback loop is essential for continuous improvement in herbal recipe development.

1. **Seeking Feedback from Users**: Encouraging those who use the herbal preparations to provide feedback on their effectiveness and any side effects.

2. **Iterative Process**: Viewing herbal recipe development as an iterative process, continually refining and improving based on feedback and new learnings.

Experimentation and adaptation in herbal medicine are not just about creating effective remedies; they represent a dynamic and interactive approach to health and wellness. By experimenting with and adapting herbal recipes, individuals can craft personalized solutions that respect traditional wisdom while embracing contemporary needs and advancements.

CALL TO ACTION FOR FURTHER HERBAL STUDY AND APPLICATION

The pursuit of knowledge is a continuous process, an ongoing commitment to learning and application. This subchapter serves as a call to action for all who are intrigued by the healing power of plants, encouraging a deeper dive into the study and practical application of herbal medicine. Here, we will explore the pathways for deepening herbal studies and ways to apply this valuable knowledge in various aspects of life and community.

The Importance of Advanced Herbal Studies

Pursuing advanced studies in herbal medicine is essential for those looking to deepen their understanding and effectiveness as herbal practitioners or enthusiasts.

1. **Deepening Herbal Knowledge**: Advanced studies provide an opportunity to delve deeper into botanical medicine, phytochemistry, and clinical applications of herbs.

2. **Specialization Opportunities**: Pursuing advanced studies allows for specialization in areas such as herbal pharmacology, women's health, pediatric herbalism, or geriatric herbalism.

Developing a Personal Herbal Philosophy

As one deepens their study in herbal medicine, developing a personal herbal philosophy becomes crucial for guiding practice and decision-making.

1. **Philosophy on Health and Healing**: Formulating a personal philosophy on health and healing that reflects one's beliefs, values, and the holistic nature of herbal medicine.

2. **Ethical Considerations**: Including ethical considerations such as sustainability, cultural respect, and patient autonomy in one's herbal philosophy.

Advocating for Herbal Medicine

As knowledge in herbal medicine grows, advocating for its rightful place in healthcare becomes a natural progression.

1. **Advocacy and Public Speaking**: Engaging in advocacy efforts, public speaking, or writing to promote the understanding and acceptance of herbal medicine in broader healthcare.

2. **Policy and Regulation Involvement**: Staying informed and involved in policy and regulation discussions related to herbal medicine to ensure fair and informed legislation that supports the practice of herbalism.

Mentorship and Teaching

Mentorship and teaching are integral parts of furthering one's journey in herbal medicine, allowing for the sharing of knowledge and experience.

1. **Seeking Mentorship**: Seeking mentors who can provide guidance, share their experiences, and offer support in advanced studies and practice.

2. **Becoming a Mentor or Teacher**: As one gains experience and knowledge, transitioning into a mentor or teacher role to guide and inspire newcomers to the field.

Documenting and Sharing Herbal Experiences

Documenting one's experiences, cases, and research findings is invaluable for personal growth and contributes to the collective knowledge in herbal medicine.

1. **Writing Articles or Blogs**: Writing articles, blogs, or case studies to document and share experiences, findings, and insights in herbal medicine.

2. **Publishing Research Findings**: For those involved in research, publishing findings in journals or online platforms to contribute to the scientific body of knowledge in herbal medicine

Personal Reflection and Self-Assessment

Regular self-reflection and assessment are crucial for personal and professional growth in the field of herbal medicine.

1. **Reflecting on Progress and Goals**: Regularly reflecting on one's progress, reassessing goals, and setting new objectives for continuous growth and development.

2. **Self-Assessment Tools**: Utilizing self-assessment tools to evaluate one's knowledge, skills, and practice, and to identify areas for improvement.

Exploring International Perspectives in Herbal Medicine

Exploring herbal medicine from an international perspective broadens one's understanding and appreciation for the field.

1. **Learning from International Traditions**: Studying herbal traditions from different parts of the world, such as Traditional Chinese Medicine, Ayurveda, or Western herbalism.

2. **Participating in International Exchanges**: Engaging in international exchanges or programs to experience different herbal practices and healthcare systems.

The call to action for further herbal study and application reiterates the need to continually expand one's knowledge, refine skills, and apply learning in meaningful ways. Through advanced studies, research, community engagement, and practical application, individuals can truly embody the essence of herbal medicine, contributing to personal wellness and the broader health of the community.

CONCLUSION OF THE BOOK

As we reach the conclusion of this enlightening journey through the world of herbal medicine and natural remedies, it is essential to pause and reflect on the profound insights and knowledge we have garnered. This book has not only been a guide to the myriad uses of herbs and their benefits but also a testament to the power of nature in healing and maintaining health. In this concluding chapter, we synthesize the key learnings, reiterate the core principles of herbal medicine, and envisage the future of this ancient yet ever-evolving practice. This is not just an end but a beacon that lights the way forward for those who seek to continue exploring the vast, verdant world of herbalism.

Synthesis of Key Learnings

Throughout this book, we have traversed various aspects of herbal medicine, from the fundamentals of herbal properties to the intricate methods of preparation and application.

1. **Holistic Understanding**: We've gained a holistic understanding of herbs; not just as mere ingredients but as entities imbued with healing properties, deeply connected to our health and the environment.

2. **Practical Knowledge**: Practical knowledge in preparing and using herbal remedies has been a key focus, empowering readers to take an active role in their health and well-being.

Reiterating Core Principles of Herbal Medicine

The core principles of herbal medicine, which have been the backbone of this book, deserve a final emphasis.

1. **Nature's Wisdom**: The principle that nature offers profound healing wisdom, and that by aligning with this wisdom, we can achieve better health and balance.

2. **Individualized Approach**: The understanding that herbal medicine is highly individualized; what works for one may not work for another, underscoring the importance of personalization in treatment.

The Role of Herbal Medicine in Modern Healthcare

In the context of modern healthcare, herbal medicine plays a complementary role, offering natural alternatives and adjuncts to conventional treatments.

1. **Integrative Approach**: The growing trend of an integrative approach to health, where herbal remedies are used alongside conventional medicine to optimize health outcomes.

2. **Preventive Healthcare**: Herbal medicine's strong emphasis on prevention, promoting wellness rather than merely treating disease.

The Future of Herbal Medicine

Looking forward, the realm of herbal medicine is poised for growth, with increasing recognition and scientific validation.

1. **Scientific Research and Validation**: The future promises more scientific research into herbal remedies, providing a stronger evidence base for their use.

2. **Global Integration:** The global integration of diverse herbal traditions, leading to a richer, more inclusive understanding of herbal medicine.

This book, in essence, is a gateway to a world where health is viewed through the lens of nature's simplicity and profundity. It invites readers to continue exploring, experimenting, and embracing the rich tapestry of herbal medicine.

Journeying through herbal medicine a path that leads to a deeper understanding of ourselves and our intrinsic connection with the natural world. As we integrate these teachings into our lives, we become part of a larger movement; one that values wellness, sustainability, and the wisdom of nature.

SUMMARIZING O'NEILL'S TEACHINGS AS INTERPRETED BY WILLOWBROOK

As we draw the curtains on this insightful exploration of herbal medicine, it is fitting to culminate by summarizing and reflecting upon the teachings of Barbara O'Neill as interpreted through the practical and intuitive lens of Margaret Willowbrook. This subchapter sublimes the essence of O'Neill's philosophy, as seen through Willowbrook's perspective, encapsulating the fundamental principles, practices, and beliefs that have shaped their approach to natural health and healing.

The Holistic View of Health

Central to O'Neill's teachings is the holistic view of health, which Willowbrook embraces and advocates. This approach considers the whole person; body, mind, and spirit, in the quest for optimal health.

1. **Interconnectedness of Body Systems**: Willowbrook echoes O'Neill's emphasis on the interconnectedness of body systems, advocating for treatments that address the underlying causes of illness rather than just symptoms.

2. **Emotional and Spiritual Health**: The recognition of emotional and spiritual factors in physical health is a key element in O'Neill's teachings, as reflected in Willowbrook's holistic practices.

Herbal Medicine and Natural Remedies

At the heart of O'Neill's teachings are herbal medicine and natural remedies, areas where Willowbrook's expertise and experience shine through.

1. **Use of Medicinal Herbs**: Willowbrook's approach reflects O'Neill's advocacy for the use of medicinal herbs, harnessing their natural healing properties for various health conditions.

2. **DIY Remedies and Self-Sufficiency**: Both practitioners emphasize the importance of preparing one's own remedies and encourage self-sufficiency in managing health.

Prevention over Treatment

The principle of prevention over treatment is a cornerstone in O'Neill's teachings, a theme consistently evident in Willowbrook's approach.

1. **Proactive Health Measures**: Emphasis on proactive measures to prevent illness, such as maintaining a healthy diet, regular exercise, and stress reduction techniques.

2. **Early Intervention**: The importance of early intervention in health issues, recognizing signs and symptoms, and addressing them naturally before they escalate, is a key tenet shared by both O'Neill and Willowbrook.

Holistic Approaches to Common Health Issues

O'Neill's approach to common health issues, which Willowbrook has adopted and adapted, involves viewing these issues through a holistic lens, considering all contributing factors.

1. **Natural Approaches to Chronic Diseases**: Methods for managing chronic diseases such as diabetes, heart disease, and arthritis using natural remedies and lifestyle changes are a focal point.

2. **Mental Health and Herbal Support**: The use of herbal remedies and lifestyle interventions to support mental health, including anxiety and depression, is a significant aspect of their teachings.

Final Thoughts and Future Directions

As Willowbrook interprets and carries forward O'Neill's teachings, she also looks to the future, considering how these principles can be adapted and expanded upon.

1. **Evolving Practices**: Recognizing that the field of herbal medicine and natural health is continually evolving, and staying abreast of new research and developments is essential.

2. **Expanding Reach and Influence**: The hope and intention to expand the reach of these teachings, influencing a broader audience to embrace natural health practices and herbal medicine.

In summarizing Barbara O'Neill's teachings through the interpretive lens of Margaret Willowbrook, we see a rich throng of holistic health principles, deeply rooted in the wisdom of nature and refined through practical application and modern understanding. These teachings go beyond mere treatments; they represent a way of life, a philosophy that intertwines health, wellness, and harmony with nature.

FINAL REFLECTIONS FROM MARGARET WILLOWBROOK, DRAWING ON O'NEILL'S WISDOM

In the concluding remarks of this comprehensive journey through the realms of herbal medicine and natural healing, Margaret Willowbrook offers her final reflections, deeply rooted in the wisdom imparted by Barbara O'Neill. This subchapter is a contemplative synthesis of the journey, encapsulating the essence of the teachings and the profound impact they have had on Willowbrook's perspective and practices. Here, Willowbrook not only reiterates the core principles she has embraced but also shares her insights on how these teachings can be integrated into our lives, shaping our approach to health, wellness, and our relationship with the natural world.

The Journey of Learning and Healing

Willowbrook begins by reflecting on her journey, a path that has been both enlightening and transformative.

1. **Personal Transformation**: She shares her experiences of personal growth and healing, attributing her profound understanding of health and wellness to the teachings of O'Neill.

2. **The Role of the Teacher**: Willowbrook emphasizes the importance of having a mentor like O'Neill, whose teachings have been instrumental in guiding her and many others on the path of natural healing.

234

Embracing Nature's Rhythms

Willowbrook's reflections bring into focus the significance of living in harmony with nature's rhythms.

1. **Seasonal Living**: She talks about the impact of aligning one's lifestyle with the changing seasons, and how this has deepened her connection with the natural world.

2. **Learning from Nature's Cycles**: Willowbrook shares insights on how observing and understanding nature's cycles can provide valuable lessons for personal health and well-being.

The Power of Simplicity

In her reflections, Willowbrook underscores the power of simplicity, a key principle she learned from O'Neill.

1. **Simplicity in Remedies**: She emphasizes the effectiveness of simple, time-tested remedies over complex formulations, advocating for the use of easily available, common herbs.

2. **Minimalism in Lifestyle**: Willowbrook also touches on the benefits of a minimalist lifestyle, reducing reliance on material things and focusing on the essentials for health and happiness.

Reflections on Personal Growth and Contribution

Willowbrook concludes with personal reflections on her growth as a practitioner and her contributions to the field.

1. **Journey of Self-Discovery**: She shares her journey of self-discovery through the study and practice of herbal medicine, describing how it has shaped her worldview and approach to life.

2. **Contribution to Community and Nature:** Willowbrook reflects on her contributions to her community and the environment, highlighting her efforts to promote sustainable practices and natural wellness.

In these final reflections, Margaret Willowbrook, inspired by the teachings of Barbara O'Neill, invites us to view our health and well-being through the lens of nature's wisdom. Her insights refine the importance of a holistic approach, the power of simplicity, and the necessity of sustainable practices in our pursuit of health. We are reminded that the journey of learning in herbal medicine is endless, filled with opportunities for growth, discovery, and deeper connection with the natural world. Willowbrook's reflections serve as a guide towards a future where natural healing is not just a practice but a way of life, deeply ingrained in our daily routines and embraced by our communities.

Important information! Why Our Book Does Not Include colored Herb Photos!

Consideration for Cost and Accessibility:
In our commitment to keeping the book affordable, we consciously decided against including color herb photos. This decision directly impacts and lowers the printing costs, making the book more accessible to a broader range of readers. Our priority is to provide comprehensive herbal knowledge at a reasonable price.

Emphasizing the Role of Visual Aids:
Understanding the importance of visual identification in herbal studies, especially for newcomers and in recipe preparation, we recommend for detailed herb images.
https://myplantin.com/plant-identifier/herb

This online resource complements our book perfectly, enabling accurate herb identification and enhancing your herbal learning experience.

OVER 300 RECIPES FOR TREATING COMMON CONDITIONS INSPIRED BY O'NEILL'S REMEDIES.

Here, we explore a collection of over 300 detailed recipes for treating common conditions. These remedies harness the natural power of herbs and are crafted with the wisdom and insight O'Neill has shared in her teachings. Organized by category for ease of reference, these recipes provide a practical guide to creating effective, natural treatments for a variety of common health issues. **For those desiring a comprehensive, step-by-step exploration of each recipe, including preparation methods, and expected outcomes, please consider acquiring Volume 2. This companion volume provides a deeper insight into each remedy, offering enriched content that complements and enhances your understanding and application of herbal medicine. With more than 440 pages, we were unable to include it in this volume, necessitating the creation of Volume 2 as a separate book. Available here:**
www.amazon.com/dp/B0CW1GT4FS

1. GENERAL HEALTH AND WELLNESS

a. Herbal Remedies for General Health and Wellness

Dandelion Root Detox Tea:
- Simmer dried dandelion root in water for 15 minutes.
- Drink to support liver detoxification.

Licorice Root Tea for Digestive Health:

- Steep dried licorice root in hot water for 10 minutes.
- Drink to support gastrointestinal health.

Nettle Tea for Allergy Relief:
- Steep dried nettle leaves in hot water for 15 minutes.
- Drink to alleviate allergy symptoms.

Dandelion Tea for Liver Detox:
- Simmer dried dandelion root and leaves in water for 15 minutes.
- Drink to support liver detoxification.

Milk Thistle Seed Extract for Liver Health:
- Take a commercially prepared milk thistle extract to promote liver health.

Cinnamon Infusion for Blood Sugar Control:
- Steep cinnamon sticks in hot water for 10 minutes.
- Drink to help regulate blood sugar levels.

Turmeric and Black Pepper Capsules for Anti-Inflammatory Benefits:
- Mix turmeric powder with a pinch of black pepper and encapsulate.
- Take capsules to harness turmeric's anti-inflammatory properties.

Lemon and Honey Sore Throat Soother:
- Mix the juice of one lemon with a tablespoon of Honey in warm water.
- Drink to soothe a sore throat.

Cinnamon and Honey Anti-Inflammatory Paste:
- Mix cinnamon powder with Honey to form a paste.
- Consume regularly for its anti-inflammatory properties.

Turmeric, Ginger, and Black Pepper Tea for Overall Wellness:
- Blend turmeric powder, ginger root, and a pinch of black pepper.
- Steep in hot water and drink for overall health benefits.

Nettle Leaf Infusion for Allergies:
- Infuse dried nettle leaves in hot water.
- Drink during allergy season for natural allergy relief.

Turmeric and Black Pepper Mix for Inflammation:
- Combine turmeric powder with a pinch of black pepper.
- Add to meals or drinks for anti-inflammatory benefits.

Nettle Leaf Tea for Allergy Relief:

- Steep dried nettle leaves in hot water.
- Drink during allergy seasons for relief.

Cinnamon and Honey Mix for Blood Sugar Control:
- Mix cinnamon powder with Honey.
- Consume regularly to help regulate blood sugar levels.

Rosehip Tea for Vitamin C Boost:
- Infuse dried rosehips in hot water.
- Drink as a natural source of vitamin C.

Lemon Balm Tea for Relaxation:
- Steep dried lemon balm leaves in hot water.
- Drink to calm nerves and promote relaxation.

Spirulina and Chlorella Smoothie for Nutritional Boost:
- Blend spirulina and chlorella powder into a smoothie.
- Consume for a rich source of vitamins and minerals.

Nettle and Horsetail Infusion for Hair Health:
- Steep nettle and horsetail in hot water.
- Drink to support hair health and strength.

Ginseng Root Tea for Energy and Vitality:
- Simmer ginseng root in water.
- Drink to enhance energy levels and overall vitality.

Elderberry and Cinnamon Syrup for Immune Support:
- Simmer elderberries and cinnamon in water, then strain.
- Add Honey to make a syrup, and take for immune support.

Rosehip and Hibiscus Tea for Vitamin C:
- Blend dried rosehips and hibiscus flowers, steep in hot water.
- Drink as a natural source of vitamin C.

Nettle and Lemon Tea for Detoxification:
- Infuse nettle leaves and a slice of lemon in hot water.
- Drink to support natural detoxification processes.

Spirulina and Wheatgrass Smoothie for Nutritional Boost:
- Blend spirulina and wheatgrass powder into a smoothie.
- Drink for a nutrient-rich boost.

Lemon and Ginger Morning Elixir for Immune Boosting:
- Mix lemon juice, grated ginger, and Honey in warm water.
- Drink in the morning to boost the immune system.

Apple cider Vinegar and Honey Tonic for Overall Wellness (Barbara do not recommend using Apple cider):
- Mix Apple cider vinegar with Honey and warm water.

- Consume daily for digestive health and general wellness.

Sea Buckthorn Berry Juice for Antioxidant Support:
- Drink sea buckthorn berry juice.
- High in antioxidants, it supports overall health and vitality.

Turmeric and Black Pepper Mix for Anti-inflammatory Benefits:
- Combine turmeric powder with a pinch of black pepper.
- Add to meals or drinks for its anti-inflammatory properties.

Siberian Ginseng (Eleuthero) Extract for Immune and Energy:
- Take Siberian ginseng extract as directed.
- Useful for boosting energy and immune system support.

Green Tea and Lemon Elixir for Antioxidant Boost:
- Mix green tea and fresh lemon juice.
- Drink regularly for its antioxidant and health-promoting properties.

Chlorella and Spirulina Powder for Detoxification:
- Blend chlorella and spirulina powder into a smoothie.
- Drink to support detoxification and nutrient intake.

Schisandra Berry Tea for Liver Health and Stress Reduction:
- Steep dried schisandra berries in hot water.

- Drink to support liver health and reduce stress.

Sea Buckthorn Berry Juice for Skin and Overall Health:
- Drink sea buckthorn berry juice.
- Rich in vitamins and antioxidants, it supports skin health and overall vitality.

Turmeric, Black Pepper, and Coconut Oil Paste for Inflammation:
- Mix turmeric powder with black pepper and coconut oil.
- Consume to utilize its anti-inflammatory and health-enhancing properties.

Moringa Leaf Powder for Nutritional Supplement:
- Mix moringa leaf powder in smoothies or water.
- Drink for its wide range of vitamins, minerals, and antioxidants.

Moringa and Wheatgrass Nutrient-Rich Blend:
- Mix moringa leaf powder with wheatgrass powder.
- Add to smoothies or water for a nutrient-dense supplement.

Astragalus and Elderberry Immune-Boosting Syrup:
- Simmer astragalus root and elderberries in water.
- Add Honey to create a syrup; consume for immune support.

Sea Moss Gel for Mineral Boost:
- Soak sea moss in water until it expands.

- Blend into a gel and consume for its rich mineral content.

Ginger and Turmeric Anti-Inflammatory Juice:
- Juice fresh ginger and turmeric roots.
- Drink to reduce inflammation and support overall health.

Stinging Nettle and Lemon Spring Detox Tea:
- Steep stinging nettle leaves and a slice of lemon in hot water.
- Drink to detoxify and refresh the body.

Chlorella and Spirulina Detox Smoothie:
- Blend chlorella and spirulina powders into a fruit smoothie.
- Consume to aid in detoxification and provide a nutrient boost.

Schisandra Berry and Licorice Root Adaptogenic Tonic:
- Mix schisandra berry extract with licorice root powder.
- Add to warm water or tea for an adaptogenic boost.

Dandelion and Burdock Root Detox Tea:
- Blend dandelion and burdock root, steep in hot water.
- Drink to support detoxification and liver health.

Senna Leaf and Fennel Seed Laxative Blend:
- Mix senna leaf and fennel seeds.

- Steep in hot water and drink to relieve occasional constipation.

Kelp and Spirulina Thyroid Support Smoothie:
- Blend kelp and spirulina into a smoothie.
- Drink to support thyroid function due to their iodine content.

Hibiscus and Rosehip Antioxidant Tea:
- Mix dried hibiscus flowers and rosehips, steep in hot water.
- Drink for a refreshing, antioxidant-rich tea.

Schisandra Berry and Goji Berry Vitality Tonic:
- Soak schisandra berries and goji berries in hot water.
- Drink to enhance overall vitality and well-being.

Lemon Balm and Mint Digestive Tea:
- Blend lemon balm and mint leaves, steep in hot water.
- Drink to soothe digestive issues and promote relaxation.

Elderflower and Yarrow Immune Boosting Tea:
- Infuse elderflower and yarrow in hot water.
- Drink at the onset of cold or flu symptoms to boost the immune system.

Dandelion and Lemon Detox Tea:
- Mix dandelion leaves with a slice of lemon in hot water.
- Drink to support liver detoxification and overall wellness.

Senna Leaf and Anise Seed Gentle Laxative Tea:
- Blend senna leaf with anise seeds.
- Steep in hot water and drink occasionally to relieve constipation.

Rosehip and Hibiscus Vitamin C Boost Tea:
- Infuse dried rosehips and hibiscus flowers in hot water.
- Drink as a natural source of vitamin C and antioxidants.

Turmeric and Black Pepper Anti-Inflammatory Blend:
- Mix turmeric powder with a pinch of black pepper.
- Add to meals or smoothies for anti-inflammatory benefits.

Astragalus Root Immune-Boosting Broth:
- Simmer astragalus root in vegetable or chicken broth.
- Consume the broth to enhance immune function.

Chia Seed and Coconut Water Hydration Mix:
- Soak chia seeds in coconut water.
- Drink to stay hydrated and energized.

Spirulina and Blueberry Superfood Smoothie:
- Blend spirulina powder with blueberries, banana, and milk of choice.
- Drink for a nutrient-rich, energizing boost.

Turmeric and Ginger Anti-Inflammatory Drink:
- Blend turmeric and ginger, add to warm water or milk.

- Drink to reduce inflammation and boost immunity.

Lemon and Ginger Detoxifying Water:
- Infuse water with fresh lemon slices and ginger.
- Drink throughout the day for detoxification and hydration.

Dandelion Green and Mint Refreshing Tea:
- Blend dandelion greens with mint leaves.
- Steep in hot water and drink for liver support and a refreshing boost.

Schisandra Berry and Licorice Root Adaptogenic Tonic:
- Mix schisandra berry powder with licorice root.
- Add to tea or warm water for an adaptogenic effect.

Elderberry and Cinnamon Immune Boosting Syrup:
- Simmer elderberries and cinnamon sticks in water, strain, and mix with Honey.
- Take a spoonful daily for immune support.

Seabuckthorn and Acai Berry Antioxidant Smoothie:
- Blend seabuckthorn and acai berry powders with fruits.
- Drink for a powerful antioxidant and nutrient-rich smoothie.

Chaga Mushroom and Cacao Health Elixir:
- Simmer chaga mushroom pieces, strain, and mix with cacao powder.
- Drink as a health-boosting elixir rich in antioxidants and minerals.

Turmeric and Black Pepper Joint Health Mix:
- Mix turmeric powder with a pinch of black pepper.
- Add to meals or drinks to support joint health and reduce inflammation.

Lemon Balm and Rose Petal Calming Tea:
- Blend lemon balm with dried rose petals.
- Infuse in hot water and drink to calm the mind and soothe the spirit.

Seaweed and Miso Soup for Thyroid Support:
- Prepare a soup with seaweed, miso, and other thyroid-supportive ingredients.
- Consume regularly for its rich iodine content and thyroid benefits.

Dandelion and Peppermint Liver Detox Tea:
- Mix dandelion root with peppermint leaves.
- Steep in hot water and drink to support liver detoxification.

Schisandra Berry and Licorice Root Adaptogenic Blend:
- Combine schisandra berry powder with licorice root.
- Add to tea or smoothies for an adaptogenic and revitalizing effect.

Chia Seed and Lemon Hydration Drink:
- Soak chia seeds in lemon-infused water.
- Drink for hydration and a rich source of omega-3 fatty acids and antioxidants.

Cinnamon and Honey Immune Booster:
- Mix cinnamon powder with Honey.
- Consume regularly to support immune health and provide antioxidant benefits.

Turmeric, Ginger, and Black Pepper Anti-inflammatory Paste:
- Combine turmeric powder, grated ginger, and black pepper with a bit of water to form a paste.
- Consume regularly to harness its anti-inflammatory effects.

Aloe vera Juice for Digestive Health:
- Drink Aloe vera juice as directed.
- Soothes the digestive tract and promotes gut health.

Spirulina and Chlorella Superfood Supplement:
- Mix spirulina and chlorella powder in water or a smoothie.
- Consume for a nutrient-rich supplement, high in vitamins and minerals.

Sea Buckthorn Berry and Rosehip Syrup for Vitamin C:
- Simmer sea buckthorn berries and rosehips in water.
- Add Honey to form a syrup; consume for its high vitamin C content and antioxidant properties.

b. Herbal Remedies for Energy and Vitality.

Ashwagandha and Licorice Root Tonic:
- Mix ashwagandha powder with a small amount of licorice root.

- Add to warm milk or water and drink to enhance energy and vitality.

Maca Root and Cacao Energy Smoothie:
- Blend maca root powder and cacao with your choice of milk and a banana.
- Drink as a nutritious energy booster.

c. Herbal Remedies for Immune Support.

Astragalus Root Decoction for Immune Boosting:
- Simmer dried astragalus root in water for 40 minutes.
- Strain and drink to strengthen the immune system.

Elderflower Tea for Respiratory Health:
- Infuse dried elderflowers in hot water for 15 minutes.
- Drink to support respiratory health, especially during colds.

Shiitake Mushroom Broth for Immune Boosting:
- Simmer shiitake mushrooms in water with herbs.
- Drink the broth to support immune function.

Astragalus and Elderberry Syrup for Immunity:
- Simmer dried astragalus root and elderberries in water.
- Add Honey to create a syrup for immune support.

Astragalus Root Soup for Immune Strengthening:
- Add astragalus root slices to soups.
- Consume for its immune-strengthening properties.

Olive Leaf Extract:
- Take commercially prepared olive leaf extract as directed.
- Useful for its immune-boosting and antiviral properties.

Reishi Mushroom Immune Elixir:
- Simmer reishi mushroom slices in water.
- Drink the decoction to boost the immune system and promote longevity.

2. MENTAL AND EMOTIONAL HEALTH

a. Herbal Remedies for Stress and Anxiety.

Ashwagandha Milk for Stress:
- Mix 1 teaspoon of ashwagandha powder in a cup of warm milk.
- Drink before bed to reduce stress.

Lemon Balm Tea for Anxiety:
- Steep dried lemon balm leaves in boiling water for 10 minutes.
- Drink as needed to alleviate anxiety.

Lavender Oil Bath for Relaxation:

- Add a few drops of lavender essential oil to a warm bath.
- Soak for relaxation and stress relief.

Holy basil (Tulsi) Tea for Stress Reduction:
- Steep dried Holy basil leaves in hot water for 10 minutes.
- Drink to reduce stress and anxiety.

Rhodiola Rosea Extract for Stress Relief:
- Take a commercially prepared rhodiola extract as directed to combat stress.

Catnip and Chamomile Relaxation Tea:
- Blend dried catnip and chamomile flowers.
- Steep in hot water for a soothing, relaxing tea.

Kava Kava Root Brew for Anxiety:
- Prepare a brew from dried kava kava root.
- Consume occasionally for its anxiety-reducing properties (note: use cautiously due to potential liver toxicity).

Ashwagandha Root Powder Mix for Stress Reduction:
- Mix ashwagandha root powder in warm milk or water.
- Drink before bed to reduce stress and improve sleep.

Scullcap and Hops Tea for Anxiety Relief:
- Blend dried scullcap and hops.
- Infuse in hot water and drink to calm anxiety and nervous tension.

Passionflower and Valerian Root Tea for Stress Relief:
- Blend dried passionflower and valerian root.
- Steep in hot water and drink to ease stress and anxiety.

Rhodiola Rosea Capsules for Adaptogenic Support:
- Take rhodiola rosea capsules as directed.
- Useful for enhancing the body's resistance to stress.

Lemon Balm and Rosemary Tea for Stress Relief:
- Blend lemon balm and rosemary, steep in hot water.
- Drink to relieve stress and uplift mood.

Hops and Lavender Sleep Pillow for Anxiety:
- Mix dried hops and lavender flowers.
- Fill a small pillow for soothing anxiety and promoting sleep.

Holy basil (Tulsi) and Chamomile Tea:
- Blend tulsi leaves and chamomile flowers.
- Infuse in hot water and drink to reduce stress and calm anxiety.

Passionflower and Lemon Balm Nighttime Tea:
- Mix dried passionflower and lemon balm.
- Steep in hot water and drink before bed to promote relaxation and sleep.

Ashwagandha and Holy basil Adrenal Support Tonic:
- Mix ashwagandha and Holy basil (tulsi) powders.
- Add to warm milk or water and drink to combat stress and adrenal fatigue.

Damiana Leaf Tea for Anxiety and Relaxation:
- Steep damiana leaves in hot water.
- Drink to ease anxiety and promote relaxation.

Lemon Verbena and Passionflower Relaxing Tea:
- Combine lemon verbena and passionflower.
- Infuse in hot water and drink to reduce stress and promote relaxation.

Withania (Ashwagandha) Root Nighttime Milk:
- Simmer withania root in milk with a touch of Honey.
- Drink before bed to alleviate stress and promote restful sleep.

St. John's Wort and Lemon Balm Tea for Mood Support:
- Mix St. John's Wort with lemon balm leaves.
- Steep in hot water and drink to alleviate mild depression and anxiety.

Rhodiola Rosea Root Extract for Stress Reduction:
- Take a commercially prepared Rhodiola Rosea extract as directed.
- Useful for combating stress and enhancing mental clarity.

Ashwagandha Root and Holy basil Tea for Stress Relief:
- Combine ashwagandha root with Holy basil (tulsi) leaves.
- Steep in hot water and drink to manage stress and anxiety.

Passionflower and Lemon Balm Nighttime Tea:

- Mix dried passionflower with lemon balm.
- Brew in hot water and drink before bedtime for relaxation.

Blue Vervain and Lavender Stress-Relief Tea:
- Blend blue vervain with lavender flowers.
- Steep in hot water and drink to reduce stress and tension.

Kava Kava Root Brew for Relaxation:
- Prepare a brew from dried kava kava root.
- Consume occasionally to relax and reduce anxiety (Note: Use cautiously due to potential liver toxicity).

Oatstraw and Lavender Tea for Nervous System Support:
- Mix oatstraw and lavender flowers.
- Infuse in hot water and drink for calming the nervous system.

b. Herbal Remedies for Mental Clarity and Focus.

Rosemary Tea for Mental Alertness:
- Steep fresh or dried rosemary leaves in hot water.
- Drink to enhance mental clarity and focus.

Ginkgo biloba Leaf Infusion for Improved Concentration:
- Infuse dried Ginkgo biloba leaves in hot water.
- Drink to support cognitive function and memory.

c. Sleep Aid And Herbal Remedies for Sleep Disorders.

Valerian Root Infusion for Insomnia:
- Steep dried valerian root in hot water for 10 minutes.
- Drink before bed to improve sleep quality.

Passionflower Nighttime Tea:
- Infuse dried passionflower in boiling water for 15 minutes.
- Drink before bedtime to aid sleep.

Hops Pillow for Deep Sleep:
- Fill a small pillow with dried hops flowers.
- Place near the head at night to promote deep sleep.

Magnolia Bark Tea for Sleep Disturbances:
- Steep magnolia bark in hot water.
- Drink before bed to promote restful sleep.

Hops and Valerian Root Pillow for Insomnia:
- Mix dried hops and valerian root.
- Fill a small pillow and place near the head at night for sleep support.

Lavender and Chamomile Sleep Sachet:
- Blend dried lavender and chamomile.
- Place in a sachet under the pillow to promote restful sleep.

Cherry and Chamomile Sleepy Time Tea:
- Blend dried cherries and chamomile flowers.
- Steep in hot water before bedtime to promote restful sleep.

Lemon Verbena and Magnolia Bark Sleep Aid:
- Mix lemon verbena leaves and magnolia bark.
- Steep in hot water and drink for sleep support.

Cherry Juice and Chamomile Sleep Aid:
- Mix cherry juice with chamomile tea.
- Drink in the evening to enhance sleep quality.

Linden Flower and Chamomile Bedtime Tea:
- Mix linden flowers and chamomile.
- Steep in hot water and drink before bed for a restful night's sleep.

Lavender and Mugwort Dream Pillow:
- Mix dried lavender and mugwort.
- Fill a small pillow to place near the head during sleep for relaxing and vivid dreams.

Lavender and Catnip Sleep Tea:
- Blend lavender flowers with catnip leaves.
- Infuse in hot water and drink before bedtime to promote restful sleep.

Poppy Seed and Honey Sleep Elixir:
- Crush poppy seeds and mix with Honey.
- Consume a small amount before bed to aid sleep.

Cherry Juice and Magnolia Bark Sleep Aid:
- Mix cherry juice with magnolia bark extract.

- Drink in the evening to support healthy sleep patterns.

Passionflower and Hop Sleep Capsules:
- Blend dried passionflower with hops.
- Encapsulate and take before bedtime for improved sleep quality.

Valerian Root and Hops Capsules for Insomnia:
- Blend powdered valerian root and hops.
- Encapsulate and take before bed to aid sleep.

Chamomile and Passionflower Tea for Restful Sleep:
- Mix chamomile and passionflower, steep in hot water.
- Drink before bedtime to promote restful sleep.

3. DIGESTIVE AND EXCRETORY SYSTEMS

a. Digestive Health Remedies.

Peppermint Tea for Indigestion:
- Boil 1 cup of water and pour over 1 teaspoon of dried peppermint leaves.
- Steep for 10 minutes, then strain.
- Drink after meals to ease indigestion.

Ginger Root Decoction for Nausea:
- Slice a 2-inch piece of fresh ginger root.
- Simmer in 2 cups of water for 15 minutes.
- Strain and sip slowly to alleviate nausea.

Fennel Seed Infusion for Bloating:
- Crush 1 tablespoon of fennel seeds.
- Steep in 1 cup of boiling water for 10 minutes.
- Drink warm to relieve bloating and gas.

Chamomile Tea for Digestive Comfort:
- Infuse dried chamomile flowers in hot water for 10 minutes.
- Drink to soothe digestive discomfort.

Slippery Elm Bark Gruel for Gastric Ulcers:
- Mix slippery elm powder with water to form a gruel.
- Consume to soothe gastric ulcers.

Slippery Elm and Marshmallow Root Tea for Gut Health:
- Mix slippery Elm bark powder and marshmallow root.
- Steep in hot water for 10 minutes and drink for digestive comfort.

Dandelion and Burdock Root Tea for Liver Detox:
- Simmer equal parts of dandelion and burdock root in water for 15 minutes.
- Drink to support liver detoxification.

Peppermint and Caraway Seed Digestive Blend:
- Mix dried peppermint leaves and caraway seeds.

- Infuse in hot water and drink after meals to aid digestion.

Peppermint and Caraway Digestive Tea:
- Mix dried peppermint leaves and caraway seeds.
- Infuse in hot water and drink after meals to aid digestion.

Milk Thistle Seed Tea for Liver Support:
- Crush milk thistle seeds and steep in hot water.
- Drink to support liver health.

Ginger and Lemon Balm Tea for Nausea:
- Blend fresh ginger and dried lemon balm.
- Steep in hot water and sip to alleviate nausea.

Artichoke Leaf Tea for Liver Health:
- Steep dried artichoke leaves in hot water.
- Drink to support liver function and bile production.

Yellow Dock Root Tea for Digestive Support:
- Simmer yellow dock root in water.
- Drink to aid digestion and liver function.

Barberry Bark Decoction for Gallbladder Health:
- Simmer dried barberry bark in water.
- Drink to support gallbladder and liver health.

Peppermint and Licorice Tea for Indigestion:
- Blend peppermint leaves and licorice root, steep in hot water.

- Drink to ease indigestion and soothe the stomach.

Marshmallow Root and Slippery Elm Bark for Gut Health:
- Mix marshmallow root and slippery Elm bark, steep in water.
- Drink to support gut health and soothe the digestive tract.

Triphala Powder for Digestive Regularity:
- Mix Triphala powder in warm water.
- Drink before bed to promote digestive regularity and detoxification.

Angelica and Peppermint Digestive Tonic:
- Blend angelica root and peppermint leaves.
- Steep in hot water and drink to aid digestion and soothe the stomach.

Fennel and Ginger Digestive Aid:
- Steep fennel seeds and fresh ginger slices in hot water.
- Drink to soothe digestive discomfort and reduce bloating.

Meadowsweet Infusion for Acid Reflux:
- Steep meadowsweet flowers in hot water.
- Drink to soothe acid reflux and protect the digestive lining.

Cardamom and Ginger Digestive Chai:
- Blend cardamom, ginger, and other chai spices.
- Boil in water and milk, and sweeten with Honey for a digestive aid.

Artichoke and Mint Digestive Tea:
- Combine dried artichoke leaves with mint.
- Steep in hot water and drink after meals for digestive support.

Slippery Elm and Marshmallow Root Soothing Gruel:
- Mix slippery Elm bark powder with marshmallow root powder and water.
- Cook to form a gruel and consume to soothe the digestive tract.

Artichoke and Mint Digestive Tea:
- Combine dried artichoke leaves with mint.
- Steep in hot water and drink after meals for digestive support.

Slippery Elm and Marshmallow Root Soothing Gruel:
- Mix slippery Elm bark powder with marshmallow root powder and water.
- Cook to form a gruel and consume to soothe the digestive tract.

Ginger and Peppermint Digestive Aid Capsules:
- Mix powdered ginger and peppermint leaves.
- Encapsulate and take after meals to aid digestion.

Chamomile and Licorice Tea for Stomach Comfort:
- Blend chamomile flowers with licorice root.
- Steep in hot water and drink to soothe the digestive tract.

Peppermint and Caraway Seed Digestive Soother:
- Mix peppermint leaves with caraway seeds.

- Steep in hot water and drink to ease digestive discomfort.

Ginger and Fennel Seed Anti-Nausea Blend:
- Combine fresh ginger slices with fennel seeds.
- Steep in hot water and sip to relieve nausea.

Slippery Elm and Marshmallow Root Soothing Tea:
- Blend slippery Elm bark with marshmallow root.
- Steep in hot water and drink to soothe and protect the digestive lining.

b. Herbal Remedies for Liver Health.

Milk Thistle Seed Decoction:
- Simmer milk thistle seeds in water for 20 minutes.
- Strain and drink to support liver detoxification and health.

Dandelion Root and Burdock Tea:
- Mix dandelion root and burdock root.
- Steep in hot water and drink to promote liver and kidney health.

c. Herbal Remedies for Kidney Health.

Parsley and Lemon Diuretic Tea:
- Steep fresh parsley and a slice of lemon in hot water.
- Drink to support kidney function and natural detoxification.

Nettle and Horsetail Kidney Support Tea:

- Blend dried nettle and horsetail.
- Infuse in hot water and drink to enhance kidney health and urinary tract function.

d. Herbal Remedies for Urinary Tract Health.

Corn silk Tea for Urinary Comfort:
- Steep dried Corn silk in hot water.
- Drink to soothe urinary tract discomfort.

Bearberry (Uva Ursi) Tea for Urinary Tract Infections:
- Infuse dried bearberry leaves in hot water.
- Drink to support urinary tract health (Note: Short-term use recommended).

Cranberry and Dandelion Tea for UTI Prevention:
- Mix dried cranberries and dandelion leaves.
- Steep in hot water and drink to support urinary tract health and prevent UTIs.

Juniper Berry and Uva Ursi Diuretic Blend:
- Blend juniper berries and uva ursi leaves.
- Steep in hot water to create a natural diuretic tea.

Bearberry Tea for Bladder Infections:
- Infuse bearberry leaves in hot water.
- Drink to help treat urinary tract and bladder infections.

Corn silk Infusion for Kidney Support:
- Steep Corn silk in boiling water.
- Drink to support kidney health and urinary function.

Cleavers and Dandelion Diuretic Infusion:
- Blend cleavers and dandelion leaves.
- Infuse in hot water and drink to support urinary tract health.

Buchu and Uva Ursi Tea for Bladder Infections:
- Mix buchu leaves with uva ursi.
- Steep in hot water and drink to alleviate bladder infections.

Juniper Berry and Parsley Seed Diuretic Blend:
- Mix juniper berries with parsley seeds.
- Steep in hot water and drink to support urinary tract function.

Horsetail and Nettle Tea for Kidney Health:
- Blend dried horsetail and nettle leaves.
- Infuse in hot water and drink to support kidney function.

Couch Grass and Corn silk Tea for UTI Relief:
- Blend dried couch grass with Corn silk.
- Infuse in hot water and drink to support urinary tract health.

Cranberry and D-Mannose Drink for Bladder Health:
- Mix cranberry juice with D-Mannose powder.
- Drink regularly to help prevent urinary tract infections.

Goldenrod and Birch Leaf Diuretic Tea:
- Mix dried goldenrod with birch leaves.
- Infuse in hot water and drink to support urinary tract health.

Cucumber and Parsley Kidney Flush Drink:
- Blend fresh cucumber with parsley and water.
- Drink to cleanse and support kidney function.

4. CARDIOVASCULAR AND RESPIRATORY SYSTEMS

a. Herbal Remedies for Cardiovascular Health.

Hawthorn Berry Tonic for Heart Health:
- Simmer dried hawthorn berries in water for 20 minutes.
- Strain and drink to support cardiovascular health.

Garlic Infusion for Blood Pressure:
- Mince fresh garlic and steep in hot water for 15 minutes.
- Strain and consume to help regulate blood pressure.

Ginkgo biloba Tea for Circulation:
- Steep dried Ginkgo biloba leaves in hot water for 10 minutes.
- Drink to promote healthy blood circulation.

Green Tea Infusion for Heart Health:
- Steep green tea leaves in hot water for 3 minutes.
- Drink regularly for its antioxidant benefits for the heart.

Garlic and Hawthorn Berry Capsules for Blood Pressure:
- Mix powdered garlic and hawthorn berry.
- Encapsulate and take daily to support healthy blood pressure.

Bilberry Tea for Circulation:
- Steep dried bilberry fruit in hot water.
- Drink regularly to support blood circulation and eye health.

Hibiscus Flower Infusion for Blood Pressure:
- Infuse dried hibiscus flowers in hot water.
- Drink daily to help manage blood pressure levels.

Cayenne Pepper Circulatory Boost Tonic:
- Mix a pinch of cayenne pepper into warm water.
- Drink to stimulate circulation and heart health.

Celery Seed Tea for Blood Pressure:
- Steep celery seeds in hot water.
- Drink regularly to support healthy blood pressure levels.

Cacao and Hawthorn Berry Heart Tonic:
- Mix powdered cacao and dried hawthorn berries.
- Steep in hot water and drink for heart health and circulation.

Flaxseed and Garlic Cholesterol-Lowering Spread:

- Grind flaxseeds and mix with crushed garlic and a bit of olive oil.
- Spread on bread or add to dishes to help lower cholesterol.

Hibiscus and Green Tea Blend for Heart Health:
- Mix dried hibiscus flowers with green tea leaves.
- Steep in hot water and drink for cardiovascular benefits.

Rose Hip and Hibiscus Heart Health Tea:
- Combine dried rose hips and hibiscus flowers.
- Steep in hot water and drink for cardiovascular benefits.

Omega-3 Rich Flaxseed Drink:
- Grind flaxseeds and mix in water or juice.
- Drink to support heart health with essential omega-3 fatty acids.

Nettle and Lemon Balm Tea for Circulation:
- Blend dried nettle leaves with lemon balm.
- Steep in hot water and drink to support circulation and heart health.

Garlic and Hawthorn Cardiovascular Tonic:
- Blend fresh garlic with hawthorn berries or extract.
- Take daily to support cardiovascular function.

b. Respiratory Health Remedies.

Thyme and Honey Cough Syrup:

- Simmer 1 tablespoon of dried thyme in 1 cup of water for 15 minutes.
- Strain and mix with equal parts Honey.
- Take 1 teaspoon as needed for cough relief.

Elderberry Syrup for Immune Support:
- Simmer dried elderberries in water for 45 minutes.
- Mash the berries, strain, and add Honey to the liquid.
- Take 1 tablespoon daily for immune support.

Mullein Leaf Tea for Respiratory Congestion:
- Infuse dried mullein leaves in boiling water for 15 minutes.
- Strain and drink to ease respiratory congestion.

Eucalyptus Steam Inhalation for Sinus Relief:
- Add a few drops of eucalyptus essential oil to a bowl of hot water.
- Inhale the steam to clear sinus congestion.

Licorice Root Decoction for Sore Throat:
- Simmer dried licorice root in water for 30 minutes.
- Drink to soothe a sore throat.

Licorice and Marshmallow Root Syrup for Cough:
- Simmer licorice and marshmallow root in water.
- Strain and mix with Honey to create a soothing cough syrup.

Mullein and Plantain Leaf Tea for Lung Support:
- o Blend dried mullein and plantain leaves.
- o Steep in hot water and drink to support lung health.

Pine Needle Steam Inhalation for Congestion:
- o Add fresh pine needles to boiling water.
- o Inhale the steam to relieve nasal and chest congestion.

Hyssop Decoction for Respiratory Relief:
- Simmer dried hyssop in water.
- Drink to relieve respiratory conditions like bronchitis.

Anise Seed Tea for Coughs:
- Steep anise seeds in boiling water.
- Drink to soothe coughs and aid expectoration.

Coltsfoot Tea for Cough Relief:
- Infuse dried coltsfoot leaves in hot water.
- Drink to soothe coughs and respiratory discomfort.

Lungwort Tea for Lung Health:
- Steep dried lungwort in hot water.
- Drink to support lung and respiratory health.

Mullein and Licorice Root Syrup for Bronchitis:
- Simmer mullein leaves and licorice root in water.
- Mix with Honey to create a syrup for respiratory relief.

Pleurisy Root Tea for Chest Congestion:
- Steep dried pleurisy root in hot water.
- Drink to relieve chest congestion and promote respiratory health.

Lobelia Inflata Extract for Asthma Relief:
- Use lobelia extract as directed for asthma relief (Note: Use under professional guidance due to its potency).

Anise and Thyme Cough Syrup:
- Simmer anise seeds and thyme in water, then mix with Honey.
- Take as needed for cough relief.

Elecampane Root Syrup for Lung Support:
- Simmer chopped elecampane root in water, then strain.
- Mix with Honey to create a syrup for respiratory health.

Pine Needle and Eucalyptus Respiratory Steam:
- Add fresh pine needles and eucalyptus leaves to boiling water.
- Inhale the steam to clear respiratory passages and ease breathing.

White Horehound Cough Syrup:
- Simmer white horehound in water, strain, and mix with Honey.
- Take as needed to soothe coughs and clear mucus.

Mint and Eucalyptus Chest Rub:

- Infuse mint and eucalyptus leaves in a carrier oil.
- Blend with beeswax to create a chest rub for respiratory relief.

Ivy Leaf Extract for Bronchial Support:
- Take ivy leaf extract as directed, especially useful for coughs and bronchial health.

Thyme and Honey Cough Syrup:
- Simmer fresh thyme in water, strain, and mix with Honey.
- Use as a natural cough syrup to soothe sore throats and coughs.

Coltsfoot and Honey Syrup for Persistent Coughs:
- Simmer coltsfoot leaves in water, strain, and mix with Honey.
- Take as needed to soothe coughs and clear mucus from the respiratory tract.

Oregano and Thyme Antimicrobial Steam:
- Add fresh oregano and thyme to boiling water.
- Inhale the steam to clear respiratory passages and combat infections.

5. MUSCULOSKELETAL AND NERVOUS SYSTEMS

a. Herbal Remedies for Pain and Inflammation.

Turmeric Golden Milk for Inflammation:
- Warm a cup of milk with 1 teaspoon of turmeric powder and a pinch of black pepper.
- Drink to reduce inflammation.

Ginger Compress for Muscle Pain:
- o Grate fresh ginger and wrap in a cloth.
- o Place in hot water, then apply the compress to sore muscles.

Willow bark Tea for Headaches:
- o Simmer dried Willow bark in water for 20 minutes.
- o Drink the tea to alleviate headache pain.

White Willow bark Decoction for Pain Relief:
- Simmer white Willow bark in water.
- Drink as a natural pain reliever for headaches and inflammation.

Boswellia Resin Extract for Joint Pain:
- Take a commercially prepared boswellia extract.
- Use for its anti-inflammatory properties, especially in joint pain.

b. Herbal Remedies for Musculoskeletal Health.

Arnica Salve for Bruises and Sprains:
- o Infuse dried arnica flowers in a carrier oil.
- o Blend with beeswax to create a salve and apply topically to bruises and sprains (Note: Do not apply to broken skin).

Comfrey Poultice for Joint Pain:
- o Make a paste from fresh comfrey leaves.
- o Apply as a poultice on sore joints for pain relief.

Epsom Salts and Lavender Bath for Muscle Relaxation:
- o Dissolve Epsom Salts in a warm bath and add a few drops of lavender essential oil.
- o Soak to relax muscles and alleviate soreness.

c. Herbal Remedies for Nervous System Health.

Bacopa Monnieri (Brahmi) Tea for Cognitive Function:
- o Steep dried Bacopa monnieri leaves in hot water.
- o Drink to enhance memory and cognitive function.

Ginkgo biloba Leaf Tea for Brain Health:
- o Infuse dried Ginkgo biloba leaves in hot water.
- o Drink to support brain health and circulation.

Gotu kola Tea for Cognitive Enhancement:
- Steep dried Gotu kola leaves in hot water.
- Drink to support memory and cognitive function.

Lemon Verbena Tea for Nervous System Support:
- Infuse dried lemon verbena leaves in hot water.
- Drink for its calming effects on the nervous system.

d. Herbal Remedies for Bone and Joint Health.

Turmeric and Ginger Tea for Joint Pain:
- Blend turmeric and ginger, steep in hot water.
- Drink to alleviate joint pain and inflammation.

Comfrey Leaf Poultice for Bone Healing:
- Make a poultice from fresh comfrey leaves.
- Apply to the affected area to aid in bone healing (Note: For external use only).

6. SPECIFIC HEALTH CONCERNS FOR MEN AND WOMEN

a. Herbal Remedies for Women's Health.

Red Clover and Sage Menopausal Support Tea:
- Blend red clover blossoms with sage leaves.
- Steep in hot water and drink for menopausal symptom relief.

Chasteberry (Vitex) and Black Cohosh Hormone Balancing Tonic:
- Mix chasteberry and black cohosh tinctures.
- Take regularly to help balance female hormones.

Black Cohosh and Sage Menopause Symptom Relief Tea:
- Blend black cohosh root with sage leaves.
- Steep in hot water and drink to alleviate menopausal symptoms.

Fenugreek Seed Lactation Booster:
- Soak fenugreek seeds in water overnight.
- Consume the seeds and water to enhance milk production in breastfeeding women.

Dong Quai and Red raspberry Leaf Tonic for Menstrual Health:
- Blend dong quai root with Red raspberry leaves.

- Steep in hot water and drink to support menstrual health.

Chaste tree (Vitex) Berry Extract for Hormonal Balance:
- Take Chaste tree berry extract as directed.
- Helpful for regulating menstrual cycles and hormonal balance.

Motherwort Tea for Menopausal Symptoms:
o Infuse dried motherwort in boiling water for 15 minutes.
o Drink to ease menopausal symptoms.

Cranberry Juice for Urinary Tract Health:
o Drink unsweetened cranberry juice regularly to maintain urinary tract health.

Evening Primrose Oil Capsules for PMS:
o Take evening primrose oil capsules as directed to alleviate PMS symptoms.

Raspberry Leaf Tea for Menstrual Cramps:
o Infuse dried raspberry leaves in hot water.
o Drink to ease menstrual cramps.

Red Clover Infusion for Menopausal Support:
o Steep dried red clover flowers in hot water.
o Drink to alleviate menopausal symptoms.

Raspberry Leaf and Nettle Tea for Pregnancy:
- o Blend dried raspberry leaves and nettle leaves.
- o Infuse in hot water and drink during pregnancy for uterine support.

Angelica Root Tea for Menstrual Support:
- Infuse dried angelica root in hot water.
- Drink to alleviate menstrual discomfort.

Fenugreek Seed Infusion for Lactation Support:
- Steep fenugreek seeds in hot water.
- Drink to enhance milk production in breastfeeding mothers.

Dong Quai and Red Clover Tea for Hormonal Balance:
- Infuse dried dong quai and red clover in hot water.
- Drink to support hormonal balance and women's health.

Vitex (Chaste tree) Berry Tea for PMS:
- Steep dried vitex berries in hot water.
- Drink to alleviate symptoms of PMS.

Cramp bark and Ginger Tea for Menstrual Cramps:
- Blend Cramp bark and fresh ginger.
- Steep in hot water and drink to relieve menstrual cramps.

Shatavari and Ashwagandha Women's Wellness Tonic:
- Mix shatavari and ashwagandha powder.
- Add to warm milk or water and drink for hormonal balance and vitality.

Evening Primrose Oil for PMS:

- Take evening primrose oil capsules as directed.
- Useful for managing PMS and menstrual discomfort.

Yarrow and Ginger Tea for Menstrual Cramps:
- Blend yarrow and ginger, steep in hot water.
- Drink to alleviate menstrual cramps.

Motherwort and Dong Quai Menstrual Relief Tonic:
- Blend motherwort and dong quai tinctures.
- Take a few drops to relieve menstrual discomfort and regulate cycles.

Raspberry Leaf and Nettle Infusion for Pregnancy:
- Steep raspberry leaf and nettle in hot water.
- Drink during pregnancy for uterine and overall women's health support.

Yarrow and Red Clover Menstrual Relief Tea:
- Combine yarrow flowers with red clover blossoms.
- Drink to alleviate menstrual discomfort and regulate the cycle.

Shatavari Root Milk for Reproductive Health:
- Simmer shatavari root in milk with a touch of Honey.
- Drink to support female reproductive health and vitality.

Evening Primrose Oil for Hormonal Balance:
- Take evening primrose oil capsules as directed.
- Helpful in managing PMS and menopausal symptoms.

b. Herbal Remedies for Men's Health.

Saw palmetto Extract for Prostate Health:
- o Take a commercially prepared Saw palmetto extract as directed.
- o Use for supporting prostate health.

Nettle Leaf Tea for Urinary Health:
- o Steep dried nettle leaves in hot water for 10 minutes.
- o Drink to support urinary tract health.

Pygeum Bark Extract for Prostate Support:
- o Take a commercially prepared pygeum extract as directed for prostate health.

Pumpkin Seed Oil for Urinary Health:
- o Consume cold-pressed pumpkin seed oil to support urinary health.

Pumpkin Seeds Snack for Prostate Health:
- o Consume raw or lightly roasted pumpkin seeds regularly for prostate health.

Pygeum Africanum Extract for Urinary Health:
- o Take a commercially prepared pygeum extract as directed for urinary health.

Uva Ursi Leaf Tea for Urinary Tract Infections:
- o Steep dried uva ursi leaves in hot water.

o Drink to support urinary tract health (note: not for long-term use).

Tribulus Terrestris Tea for Libido:
o Steep dried Tribulus terrestris in hot water.
o Drink to support male libido and vitality.

Saw palmetto Berry Tea for Prostate Health:
o Infuse dried Saw palmetto berries in hot water.
o Drink to support prostate health.

Lycopene-rich Tomato Juice for Prostate Health:
• Drink freshly made tomato juice, rich in lycopene.
• Consume regularly for prostate health support.

Zinc-rich Pumpkin Seed Snack for Male Fertility:
• Eat raw or roasted pumpkin seeds as a snack.
• Provides zinc, beneficial for male fertility and prostate health.

Pygeum Bark Extract for Prostate Support:
o Take a commercially prepared pygeum extract as directed for prostate health.

Pumpkin Seed and Saw palmetto Blend for Prostate Health:
• Mix ground pumpkin seeds with Saw palmetto extract.
• Consume regularly to support prostate health.

Nettle Root Extract for Male Vitality:
• Take nettle root extract as directed.

- Useful for supporting overall male vitality and health.

Maca Root Powder for Male Energy and Libido:
- Mix maca root powder in smoothies or water.
- Consume for increased energy and libido support.

Saw palmetto and Pygeum Africanum Extract for Prostate Health:
- Take commercially prepared extracts as directed.
- Supports prostate health and urinary function.

Pumpkin Seed Oil for Prostate and Urinary Health:
- Consume cold-pressed pumpkin seed oil regularly.
- Beneficial for prostate health and urinary tract function.

Flaxseed and Pumpkin Seed Prostate Health Smoothie:
- Blend flaxseeds and pumpkin seeds into a smoothie.
- Consume regularly to support prostate health.

Ginseng and Ginkgo biloba Tonic for Male Vitality:
- Mix ginseng and Ginkgo biloba extracts.
- Take as directed to enhance vitality and cognitive function.

Epimedium (Horny Goat Weed) and Maca Libido Booster:
- Blend powdered epimedium with maca root powder.

- Add to smoothies or drinks to enhance libido and energy.

Green Tea and Pumpkin Seed Prostate Health Blend:
- Mix green tea leaves with ground pumpkin seeds.
- Steep in hot water and drink to support prostate health.

Lycopene-rich Tomato Juice for Prostate Health:
- Drink fresh tomato juice, rich in lycopene.
- Beneficial for maintaining prostate health.

Epimedium (Horny Goat Weed) Tea for Libido Enhancement:
- Steep dried Epimedium leaves in hot water.
- Drink to naturally boost libido and sexual health.

Saw palmetto and Nettle Root Extract for Prostate Health:
- Take Saw palmetto and nettle root extract as directed.
- Supports prostate health and urinary function.

Pomegranate Juice for Antioxidant Support:
- Drink pomegranate juice regularly.
- Rich in antioxidants, it's beneficial for overall men's health.

Tribulus Terrestris and Zinc Tonic for Male Vitality:
- Blend Tribulus Terrestris extract with zinc-rich foods or supplements.
- Consume to support male vitality and overall health.

Fenugreek Seed Tea for Men's Health:
- Steep fenugreek seeds in hot water.
- Drink to support testosterone levels and men's health.

Ginseng Tea for Vitality:
- Steep ginseng root in hot water.
- Drink to enhance overall vitality and energy.

Zinc-rich Herbal Mix for Male Health:
- Combine pumpkin seeds, watermelon seeds, and sunflower seeds.
- Consume regularly for their zinc content, beneficial for male health.

7. EXTERNAL BODY HEALTH AND CARE

a. Herbal Remedies for Skin Health and Care.

Calendula Salve for Eczema:
- Infuse dried calendula petals in olive oil for 2 weeks.
- Strain and mix with melted beeswax to form a salve.
- Apply to affected areas for eczema relief.

Aloe vera Gel for Sunburn:
- Extract the gel from an Aloe vera leaf.
- Apply directly to the sunburnt skin for soothing relief.

Tea Tree Oil Blend for Acne:

- o   Mix 1 part Tea tree oil with 9 parts water.
- o   Apply to acne spots with a cotton ball.

Plantain Leaf Poultice for Skin Irritations:
- o   Crush fresh plantain leaves to release their juice.
- o   Apply as a poultice to soothe skin irritations.

Yarrow Compress for Wound Healing:
- o   Steep dried yarrow in hot water for 15 minutes.
- o   Soak a cloth in the liquid and apply to wounds.

Burdock Root Infusion for Acne:
- o   Simmer dried burdock root in water for 30 minutes.
- o   Drink to help clear acne from within.

Calendula Infused Oil for Skin Irritations:
- o   Infuse dried calendula flowers in a carrier oil.
- o   Apply the oil to soothe skin irritations and rashes.

Tea Tree Oil Spot Treatment for Acne:
- o   Dilute Tea tree oil with water or a carrier oil.
- o   Apply directly to acne spots with a cotton swab.

Oatmeal and Chamomile Bath for Eczema:
- o   Blend oatmeal and chamomile flowers.
- o   Add to a bath to soothe eczema and irritated skin.

Witch hazel and Lavender Skin Toner:

- o Mix Witch hazel extract with a few drops of lavender essential oil.
- o Apply to the skin as a natural toner for acne and inflammation.

Comfrey Salve for Wound Healing:
- o Infuse comfrey leaves in oil.
- o Mix with beeswax to create a salve and apply to wounds and bruises.

Chickweed Ointment for Itchy Skin:
- o Infuse chickweed in oil.
- o Combine with beeswax to form an ointment for itchy and irritated skin.

Burdock Root Tea for Skin Detoxification:
- Simmer dried burdock root in water.
- Drink to help detoxify the skin and improve complexion.

Chickweed Infused Oil for Itchy Skin:
- Infuse dried chickweed in a carrier oil.
- Apply to itchy, irritated skin for relief.

Witch hazel and Aloe vera Gel for Skin Irritations:
- Mix Witch hazel extract with Aloe vera gel.
- Apply to the skin for soothing and healing properties.

Neem Leaf Paste for Acne and Eczema:
- Make a paste from neem leaf powder and water.
- Apply to affected areas for skin healing benefits.

Witch hazel and Calendula Acne Treatment:
- Mix Witch hazel extract with calendula-infused oil.
- Apply to acne-prone areas for soothing and healing.

Plantain Leaf and Yarrow Wound Salve:
- Infuse plantain leaves and yarrow in a carrier oil.
- Blend with beeswax to create a salve for cuts and wounds.

Calendula and Honey Healing Ointment:
- Infuse calendula in a carrier oil, then blend with beeswax and Honey.
- Apply to skin to promote healing and soothe irritations.

Tea Tree and Witch hazel Acne Solution:
- Dilute Tea tree oil with Witch hazel.
- Apply to acne-prone areas for its antimicrobial benefits.

Comfrey and Plantain Leaf Healing Balm:
- Infuse comfrey and plantain leaves in a carrier oil, then blend with beeswax.
- Apply to minor cuts and skin irritations for healing.

Borage Seed Oil for Dermatitis and Eczema:
- Apply borage seed oil topically to affected areas.
- Useful for treating dermatitis and eczema due to its gamma-linolenic acid content.

Calendula and Chamomile Skin Soothing Lotion:
- Infuse calendula and chamomile in a carrier oil.
- Blend with Aloe vera gel to create a soothing skin lotion.

Comfrey Leaf and Plantain Skin Healing Salve:
- Infuse comfrey leaves and plantain in a carrier oil.
- Blend with beeswax to create a salve for skin healing and irritation relief.

Green Tea and Honey Facial Tonic for Acne:
- Infuse green tea, cool, and mix with Honey.
- Apply to the face as a tonic for acne-prone skin.

Aloe vera and Calendula Gel for Sunburn:
- Mix Aloe vera gel with calendula-infused oil.
- Apply to sunburnt skin for soothing relief.

Yarrow and Witch hazel Skin Toner:
- Infuse yarrow and Witch hazel bark in water.
- Apply to the skin as a toner for its astringent and healing properties.

Borage and Flaxseed Oil Eczema Relief Blend:
- Mix borage oil with flaxseed oil.
- Apply topically to soothe eczema and improve skin health.

Aloe vera and Calendula Gel for Skin Healing:
- Mix Aloe vera gel with calendula-infused oil.
- Apply to the skin for soothing and healing properties.

Nettle Leaf and Rosemary Hair Rinse for Scalp Health:

- Steep nettle leaves and rosemary in hot water.
- Use as a hair rinse to promote scalp health and hair growth.

Burdock Root and Nettle Skin Clearing Tea:
- Mix burdock root with nettle leaves.
- Steep in hot water and drink to support skin health and clarity.

Comfrey and Honey Wound Healing Ointment:
- Blend comfrey leaf-infused oil with beeswax and Honey.
- Apply to minor wounds and cuts for accelerated healing.

b. Herbal Remedies for Hair and Scalp Health.

Rosemary and Nettle Hair Rinse for Hair Growth:
- Steep rosemary and nettle leaves in boiling water.
- Use as a final rinse after shampooing to promote hair growth.

Horsetail Silica Rinse for Hair Strengthening:
- Infuse horsetail in hot water.
- Use as a hair rinse to strengthen hair, thanks to its high silica content.

c. Herbal Remedies for Eye Health.

Bilberry Extract for Vision Support:
- Take a commercially prepared bilberry extract as directed.
- Useful for supporting healthy vision and eye health.

Eyebright Tea for Eye Strain:
- Steep dried eyebright herb in hot water.
- Use as an eyewash or drink for relieving eye strain and irritation.

Eyebright and Chamomile Eye Wash for Eye Strain:
- Infuse eyebright and chamomile in boiled water.
- Use as an eye wash to relieve eye strain and irritation.

Bilberry and Goji Berry Tea for Vision Support:
- Steep dried bilberries and goji berries in hot water.
- Drink to support eye health and vision.

d. Herbal Remedies for Oral Health.

Clove and Myrrh Mouthwash for Oral Hygiene:
- Infuse clove and myrrh in water.
- Use as a mouthwash to maintain oral health and alleviate toothache.

Sage and Sea Salt Gargle for Sore Throats:
- Mix sage infusion with sea salt.
- Gargle to soothe sore throats and oral inflammations.

For those desiring a comprehensive, step-by-step exploration of each recipe, including preparation methods and expected outcomes, please consider acquiring Volume 2. This companion volume provides a deeper insight into each remedy, offering enriched content that complements and enhances your understanding and application of herbal medicine. With more than 440 pages, we were unable to include it in this volume, necessitating the creation of Volume 2 as a separate book. Available here:

www.amazon.com/dp/B0CW1GT4FS

LAST WORDS

As we reach the conclusion of this journey through the world of herbal remedies, I want to extend my heartfelt congratulations and gratitude to you, the reader, for embarking on this path of natural healing and holistic wellness. Your commitment to exploring and embracing the wisdom encapsulated in these pages is not only commendable but a vital step towards a more harmonious and balanced way of life.

This book, inspired by the teachings of Barbara O'Neill and the timeless wisdom of herbal medicine, is more than just a collection of recipes; it is a testament to the power of nature in healing and nurturing our bodies and minds. Each remedy, carefully crafted and detailed, is a drop in the vast ocean of natural healing practices that humanity has cultivated over millennia.

As you close this book, remember that it is not meant to be tucked away and forgotten. Let it be a living resource, a companion in your ongoing journey towards wellness. Keep it within reach, for the wisdom it contains is meant to be revisited, whether to find a remedy for a specific ailment or to seek inspiration for maintaining daily health and vitality.

The world of herbal medicine is dynamic and ever evolving, and so should be your relationship with these remedies. Feel encouraged to adapt and tailor these recipes to suit your unique needs and circumstances. Listen to your body, for it speaks a language older than any text, guiding you towards the herbs and preparations that resonate most with your personal journey to health.

Remember, each step you take in incorporating these natural remedies into your life is a step towards a deeper connection with the natural world and a more profound understanding of

293

your own body. The path to wellness is as much about nurturing the spirit and mind as it is about healing the body.

In closing, let this book be a gateway to an empowered and informed approach to health, one where you are the custodian of your well-being, guided by the gentle yet powerful wisdom of nature. Congratulations once again on completing this book, and may your journey through the art of herbal remedies be enriching, enlightening, and full of health and happiness.

With warm regards and best wishes for your continued health and wellness,

Margaret Willowbrook.

INDEX

REFERENCES

1. **"The Herbal Apothecary: 100 Medicinal Herbs and How to Use Them"** by JJ Pursell (2015)
2. **"The Herbal Medicine-Maker's Handbook: A Home Manual"** by James Green (2000)
3. **"Making Plant Medicine"** by Richo Cech (2000)
4. **"The Complete Herbal Tutor"** by Anne McIntyre (2010)
5. **"Rosemary Gladstar's Medicinal Herbs: A Beginner's Guide"** by Rosemary Gladstar (2012)
6. **"Back To Eden"** by Jethro Kloss (1939)
7. **"Common Herbs for Natural Health"** by Juliette de Bairacli Levy (1974)
8. **"Complete Earth Medicine Handbook"** by Susanne Fischer-Rizzi (1996)
9. **"Herbal: 100 Herbs from the World's Healing Traditions"** by Mimi Prunella Hernandez (2021)
10. **"The Way of Herbs"** by Michael Tierra (1998)
11. **"Alchemy of Herbs"** by Rosalee de la Forêt (2017)
12. **"Herbal Recipes for Vibrant Health"** by Rosemary Gladstar (2008)
13. **Books and lectures** from Barbara O'Neill.

A MESSAGE FROM THE PUBLISHER:

Are you enjoying the book? We would love to hear your thoughts!

Many readers do not know how hard reviews are to come by and how much they help a publisher. We would be incredibly grateful if you could take just a few seconds to write a brief review on Amazon, even if it's just a few sentences!

Please be aware that this is an ongoing project, and we are continuously improving the book's content thanks to your feedback. While it may not be perfect yet, your support greatly helps us!

Please go here to leave a quick review:

https://amazon.com/review/create-review?&asin=B0CSW1355L

We would greatly appreciate it if you could take the time to post your review of the book and share your thoughts with the community. If you have enjoyed the book, please let us know what you loved the most about it and if you would recommend it to others. Your feedback is valuable to us, and it helps us to improve our services and continue to offer high-quality literature to our readers.

Unlock the Next Chapter of Herbal Mastery with Volume 2

As you near the conclusion of this transformative journey through Volume 1, we invite you to delve deeper into the art and science of herbal healing with the forthcoming Volume 2. Building upon the foundational principles and broader concepts introduced here, Volume 2 offers an unparalleled exploration into the practical application of herbal wisdom for various health concerns.

Why Volume 2 Is an Essential Addition to Your Wellness Library:

- Deep Dive into Herbal Remedies: Explore the specifics of each remedy with comprehensive descriptions that go beyond Volume 1, offering a depth of knowledge that is both rare and invaluable.
- Practical, Actionable Guidance: With its focus on the practical application of herbal knowledge, Volume 2 serves as a hands-on manual for those looking to apply these healing techniques in their everyday lives.
- Empowerment Through Education: This volume empowers you with a detailed understanding of the healing powers of herbs, enabling you to enhance your health and well-being naturally.

Continue Your Journey Into Herbal Healing:
Don't let your journey end here. Volume 2 awaits to take you further into the world of natural wellness, where ancient wisdom meets modern needs. Whether you're a seasoned herbalist or a curious newcomer, this book is a must-have for anyone serious about harnessing the power of nature for health and healing.

Secure Your Copy of Volume 2 Today:
Ready to expand your herbal knowledge and continue your journey into natural healing? Click the link below to secure your copy of Volume 2. Embrace this opportunity to deepen your connection with nature's bounty and elevate your practice of herbal medicine.

Continue Your Herbal Healing Journey with Volume 2
Available here:
https://www.amazon.com/dp/B0CW1GT4FS

87031932R00174